# HEAL YOUR BACK

# HEAL YOUR BACK

Your Complete Prescription
for Preventing, Treating,
and Eliminating Back Pain

David Borenstein, M.D.

M. Evans

*Lanham · New York · Boulder · Toronto · Plymouth, UK*

ATTENTION: This book includes the most up-to-date information about conventional and complementary therapy for low back pain, based upon my thirty-two years of clinical experience with people with spine problems. The object of this book is to educate people about low back pain and offer relief of this disorder. Despite these good intentions, this book cannot offer any guarantee about the ultimate resolution of your back condition. Do not be tempted to use this book as a substitute for a medical evaluation. An examination by a health professional is always an appropriate approach to the evaluation of low back pain. Your physician has the unique advantage of listening to your description of your problem and completing a physical examination before forming an opinion about the cause of your back pain. The information in this book may differ from the advice offered by your health care provider. The recommendations in this book are not meant to replace medical treatment or diagnosis by your physician. When in doubt about the advice you have received, obtain a second opinion from another health care professional. Ultimately, you are solely responsible for your own medical decisions.

Published by M. Evans
An imprint of The Rowman & Littlefield Publishing Group, Inc.
4501 Forbes Boulevard, Suite 200, Lanham, Maryland 20706
http://www.rlpgtrade.com

Estover Road, Plymouth PL6 7PY, United Kingdom

Distributed by National Book Network

British Library Cataloguing in Publication Information Available

Library of Congress Cataloging-in-Publication Data
Borenstein, David G.
  Heal your back : your complete prescription for preventing, treating, and eliminating back pain / David Borenstein.
    p. cm.
  Includes bibliographical references and index.
  ISBN 978-1-59077-185-3 (pbk. : alk. paper) — ISBN 978-1-59077-186-0 (electronic : alk. paper)
  1. Backache—Popular works. 2. Backache—Treatment—Popular works. 3. Backache—Prevention—Popular works. I. Title.
  RD771.B217B6695 2011
  617.5'64—dc22

                                                                2010037696

Printed in the United States of America

*This book is dedicated to all my patients
who have given me the honor of being their physician.
This work is the result of their persistent requests
to put my explanations of their back problems on paper.*

# Contents

# Acknowledgments

I WANT TO THANK the individuals who have been willing to lend support, encouragement, and expertise in the development and review of this book:

Arthur Frank, M.D., medical director of the Weight Management program at the George Washington University Medical Center, for his thoughtful comments concerning the food and nutrition sections of this book.

John Starr, M.D., orthopedic surgeon, for offering his expertise in reviewing the surgical components of this book.

Tom Welsh, R.P.T., physical therapist, for his generosity and friendship in allowing his exercise program to be included in this book.

Nancy Love, my literary agent, for having confidence in me and finding a company to publish my book.

Marian Betancourt, my current literary agent, for representing me after the untimely passing of Nancy Love.

Judy Guenther, illustrator, for taking my ideas and drawing illustrations that make understanding much easier.

Rick Rinehart, my editor, for making this new volume possible.

My partners at Arthritis and Rheumatism Associates—David Wolfe, M.D.; Shari Diamond, M.D.; Angus Worthing, M.D.; Robert Lloyd, M.D., Herbert Baraf, M.D.; Robert Rosenberg, M.D.; Evan Siegel, M.D.; Emma DiIorio, M.D.; Alan Matsumoto, M.D.; Paul DeMarco, M.D.; and Ashley Beall, M.D.—for being supportive and understanding during the development and production of this book.

# Introduction

## *One Big Sneeze Can Do You In*
## *and the Twist and Shout*

I KNEW BETTER than to bend over to grab a pair of socks from the bottom drawer—that was my first mistake. I knew I should bend my knees and reach down, rather than bending "in half." Twisting from the waist was my second mistake, although I had used that motion thousands of times and it had never affected me the way it did now. Just as I started to straighten up, I felt a sharp pain on the right side of my back as the muscles there went into spasm. The pain was like a knife cut—it literally took my breath away, and I couldn't move.

Rational thinking and severe pain do not go hand in hand. In fact, when one is in pain, the most ridiculous thoughts seem perfectly reasonable. Bracing myself against the dresser that morning, I began to consider how I would put my clothes on without feeling the excruciating pain in my back. The socks in my hands seemed miles away from my feet, so how would I ever get them on? Limping as I put one foot in front of the other, bracing against the furniture for support, I began to gather up other clothes, being careful to test each small motion to see if it would bring on more pain. Putting on my shirt wasn't so bad, but I couldn't imagine how I would get my pants on. So maybe I could just show up at the office without them. Perhaps the staff wouldn't even notice!

I felt like a prisoner in my body, stuck in one place, in one position. I tried to straighten up a couple of times before I was successful, but my back was stiff and it took great effort. As if I didn't have enough going on, a big sneeze "exploded" before I could prevent it—and the spontaneous body movements that came with it. I had thought my pain was a

10 on a ten-point scale, but I was wrong. The sneeze shot me up to 14 or 15 for at least a few seconds. In addition to the increased intensity of the pain, it was now spreading up and down my back. After the second sneeze, I thought I was going to die.

Eventually, I managed to work up the courage to complete a series of "bracing and bending" movements, and carefully using the handrail on the stairway, I limped down to face breakfast, which I ate standing up. Then I took a couple of pain relievers, hoping that as the day continued my range of motion would improve. Bending over the sink to brush my teeth was out of the question, so I accomplished that task with a towel around my collar and a plastic cup of water.

Driving to my office wasn't so bad—once I had eased myself into the car. As I drove along, I did my best to avoid potholes, which looked deeper than ever. So far, every small decision, every normally routine and insignificant task, required careful consideration. Pain and restricted motion led me to park the car in a place where no neighboring cars would limit how far I could swing my door open, because it would be a chore to get out of the car. With my back straight, I moved my legs around and held on while I stood up. Normally, I get some extra exercise by walking up the stairs to my office, but today, the elevator looked very inviting.

Pain turned my usually comfortable office into a minefield. I had to maneuver around chairs and file cabinets and desks. And the biggest mine in the field was, of all things, my soft cushion recliner. I knew a firmer chair with less give was a much better choice. Throughout the day I continued to make one small choice after another to accommodate the pain and discomfort. For example, I avoided twisting my body to see the computer screen, I carried only two files at a time, and I changed position often in order to avoid becoming stuck in one place. It goes without saying that I canceled my scheduled exercise session with my workout partner.

Pain relievers helped dull the pain throughout the day, and I was able to see my patients without outwardly looking like a patient myself. But all my "extra" tasks—article research, notes to patients or doctors, letters to sign, and so forth—were put aside for another day. There is nothing like back pain to put one's priorities in place.

Even though it took longer, I took a route home that seemed "safer," because it had fewer obstacles and potholes. All this concern and conscious thought about my pain and moving my body was exhausting.

Pain is a major stressor, and I wasn't surprised that I was so tired. Eating dinner hardly seemed worth the effort, but if I wanted to take more painkillers, and I did, then I needed to eat.

Standing in the shower and letting the hot water run down my back for a few minutes allowed me to carefully bend and stretch the muscles, which restored some range of motion. I moved slowly, letting the pain guide how far I could bend. This experiment in motion didn't last long, and I didn't move very far, but I would try again tomorrow.

Sleep is always a concern when one is in pain. Getting into bed, which involved lowering my upper back with the help of my arms while at the same time raising my legs, triggered more shots of pain. But at least I was there. I stayed on my back and bent my knees over a pillow. As I drifted off to sleep, I tried to remember what got me into this fix in the first place. Of course—the blasted socks!

I thought I had learned my lesson from my first severe episode of low back pain. It had been years since my back had bothered me. I had a **magnetic resonance imaging (MRI)** test as part of a study showing changes appropriate for my age. I enjoyed playing racquet sports on a regular basis. Aerobic exercise was good training for the cardiovascular system and the stretching afterward helped my flexibility, or so I thought.

I was doing well at my game of racquet sports that afternoon. I had won two games out of three. I was warmed up and feeling good. My opponent hit the ball into the corner, just beyond my reach. Instinctively, I ran to the ball twisting my rib cage as I approached the corner of the court. I started to turn and realized that I had rotated further around than I had all game long. I could feel the muscles in my back start to tighten. I had compressed the two sides of the facet joint on the right side of my low back too much. I had had that awful feeling before when I had back pain reaching for my socks from the bottom drawer of my dresser. I foolishly thought it would not be too bad. I was warmed up. I had not really rotated that far. However, as I started to untwist my back, I knew I was wrong. I let out a shout as the entire lower portion of my back stiffened up. I could hardly move; I looked at my friend and told him he had won. I was going to stop playing now and get back to him when I would be ready to play again, probably in four weeks.

I had irritated one of the joints in my low back. In reaction, the surrounding muscles had contracted to protect the joint. My body did not want any extra movement around this joint. Gradually, the muscles loosened as the **anti-inflammatory** drug I was taking stated to calm the local inflammation inside the irritated joint. I followed my own advice to keep moving. What worked for the patients should also work for me. Some of my patients noted that I was sitting straighter in my chair when I was speaking with them. Some did not mind that I was standing during some of my interviews with them. I tried not to sit in any one place for long periods of time.

I started to do my flexion exercises to stretch my back muscles. I made sure not to twist my back as I did these exercises. Over the next three weeks, the pain and stiffness in my back improved. I could sit and stand without pain but I was not ready to return to the court. I had to wait six weeks before I was ready to hit the ball again. I did my stretching exercises before I started to play. I did some rotations of my spine to be sure that my spine was ready. I promised myself that I would not be caught with another "Twist and Shout" situation again. I would rather have my opponent win the point.

Back pain will ruin any day, and it has certainly ruined a few of mine. That's why I wrote this book, not only because I've been treating my patients for back pain, but because my own pain has given me the kinds of insights that helped me develop my basic back pain relief and ABC prevention plan.

Every second, two Americans develop low back pain. Each year 50 million of us suffer episodes of low back pain. If you are reading this book, you have experienced back pain—you may be in pain right now. Low back pain can begin with something as seemingly trivial as a sneeze, a cough, a simple twisting motion, or even bending over to grab a pair of socks. Or it can be a symptom of a more serious disease.

The men and women who arrive in my office have diverse backgrounds, careers, and lifestyles, but they all share a common complaint. They have sore, aching backs, and the pain almost always interferes with their lives. These patients have something else in common. To one degree or another, they are afraid. Most people are misinformed about both the causes of their pain and the treatments available to solve their problems. This lack of information feeds the fear that hinders recovery. Some people are afraid that they will be unable to work, while others fear their pain is a symptom of a dread disease such as cancer. Some women are concerned about their ability to carry a pregnancy; others want to prevent the progression of a spinal deformity that occurred in a close relative.

Almost all my patients arrive with questions. What can they do to improve their condition? Should they exercise? Will yoga or tai chi help? Would manipulation "straighten" a crooked spine, relieve musculoskeletal pain, and, best of all, leave them pain-free?

The best way to read this book is from the beginning, because the more you know about how your back works and the reasons why it hurts, the easier it will be to correctly diagnose and relieve your pain. You will learn how to tell whether your pain is mechanical or medical; that is, related to a problem with the dynamics of your musculoskeletal system, or related to a systemic cause like **nerve** damage from diabetes. I will show you how my basic back pain relief program can help most back pain; how you can work with your doctor to correctly diagnose and treat back pain; and how and when to use drugs, exercise, and even complementary therapies such as relaxation techniques.

Many people let back pain prevent them from doing the things they love, and this is one of the saddest results of back pain. With my book you will learn how to get into and out of bed without hurting your back, and also—and very important—how to enjoy sex without hurting your back. In the back of the book you will find many resources for more information, as well as my Back School FAQ, which comes from the questions my patients most frequently ask me.

But the most important message I can bring you is that you are in control. You can prevent episodes of back pain by following the ABC plan. If, despite your best efforts, you have a back pain, the more you learn about how your back works and why it hurts, the better your chances at finding relief. When people don't follow through with a doctor's prescription for their pain, it is most often because they don't really understand how the remedy is supposed to work, or how their body works. I hope this book will help you develop your own unique prescription for back pain relief, and put you back in control.

Now, I am going to take my own advice and put my socks in the top dresser drawer.

**Boldface words appear in the glossary.**

# Part I

# TAKING THE MYSTERY OUT
# OF LOW BACK PAIN

# Chapter 1

# Understanding Why Your Back Hurts

WHEN YOUR BACK HURTS, you feel quite alone. You think that no one can understand the extent of your discomfort. However, **low back** pain is the second most common affliction of humankind; only the common cold affects more people. Back pain doesn't discriminate, either. People of all ages, both sexes, and all walks of life are afflicted with this debilitating discomfort. Perhaps you are a computer operator who sits at a desk for hours at a time, or maybe you're a farmer or construction worker who engages in heavy lifting every day. If you happen to be a pregnant woman, then you may have difficulty finding any comfortable position—standing or sitting or lying flat on your back.

If you lift, bend, reach, squat, twist, or turn—or even sneeze—you are at some risk for developing back pain. In addition, a variety of medical conditions can result in back pain. So, as you can see, all six or so billion of us are vulnerable to back pain. In fact, it is documented that almost 80 percent of the human population will experience back pain at some point in their lives.

## IS IT MECHANICAL OR MEDICAL?

Low back pain is a form of rheumatism. **Rheumatism** is any type of problem in the musculoskeletal system. Most low back pain results from mechanical disorders of the spine related to overuse, such as habitually poor posture, or injury or deformity of a portion of the spine, such as **herniated disc**. The other 10 to 15 percent of cases are medical, caused by systemic illnesses such as **nerve** damage from diabetes or **fibromyalgia**, and require a more complete evaluation. I refer to this form of back pain as medical low back pain.

Discomfort associated with specific causes of low back pain has reproducible characteristics. For instance, ruptured discs pressing on nerves cause pain that runs from the back to the lower leg and foot. The pain from **muscle** injuries in the back may spread across the low back but not lower than the buttock. Knowing where the pain initially starts and ends helps us make a good guess about the cause.

Mechanical disorders are caused by local problems in the bones, **joints**, **tendons**, **ligaments**, muscles, and nerves of the low back. Characteristically, being active or at rest has an effect on the intensity of the pain, either making it better or worse. The position of the spine also affects the degree of pain. If you have a disc herniation, you feel more pain when you sit, while people with spinal **arthritis** feel worse when standing. Most mechanical problems heal or improve with time, physical therapy, and medications. Only 1 to 2 percent of these mechanical difficulties call for surgical intervention, such as when they cause loss of bladder control or leg weakness.

Medical disorders cause symptoms throughout the body and are not limited to discomfort in the **lumbar** spine, and they don't get better or worse with activity or rest. In addition, many organs such as the kidneys, bladder, gastrointestinal system, lymph nodes, and major blood vessels fit up against the lower back (see fig. 1.1). Diseases that affect these organs can cause back pain, with each organ system causing a certain kind of pain. When back pain originates in a structure other than the spine, the unique character of the pain can help doctors find the diseased organ system.

Medical disorders generally produce these "red flags":

- Fever and/or weight loss
- Pain that is worse at night or when lying down
- Prolonged morning stiffness lasting hours
- Severe bone pain in the middle of the back
- Pain associated with eating, urination, or the menstrual cycle

If you have any of these symptoms, see your doctor to find out if a systemic illness is causing your low back pain.

And while trauma to your back is mechanical, there are times when it becomes an emergency. Direct trauma to the lumbar spine may cause pain in any location in the low back, lower leg, or anterior thigh. These traumas are frequently the result of automobile accidents or falls. If

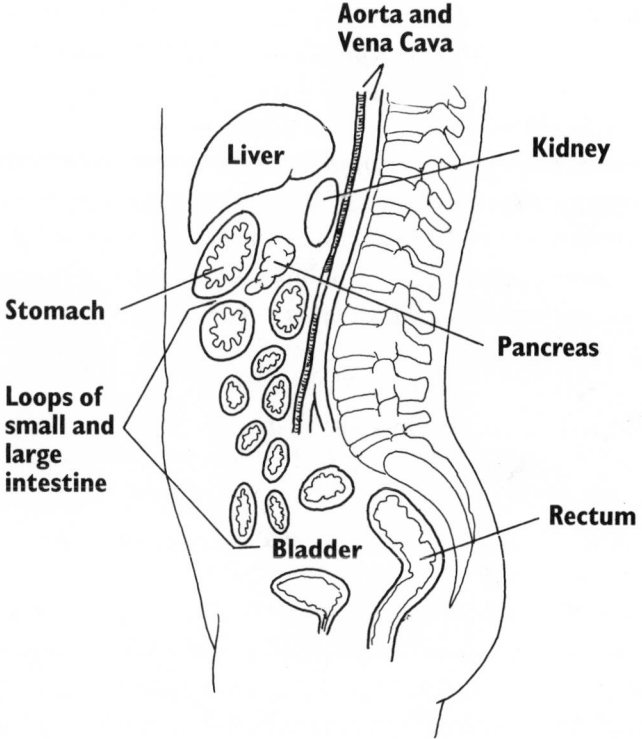

Figure 1.1.    This side view shows the major organs and blood vessels near the lumbar spine.

the trauma is severe, emergency surgery may be needed to stabilize the spine and remove pressure on the nerves. Fractures of **vertebrae** without nerve compression generally call for bracing and rest. Lesser traumas to muscles and ligaments may be treated with medications and physical therapy.

Mary is an example of how medical and mechanical causes of back pain can be confused. Mary loved to work in her garden; and although at sixty-five she had occasional aches and pains after a long day of weeding and pruning, her discomfort disappeared in a day or two. However, one day she tripped and fell backward, landing on her behind. The fall caused acute discomfort that she brushed off at the time, but over the following three weeks the pain in the middle of her back increased in intensity, making it increasingly difficult to work in her garden. When she came to see me, Mary still believed her pain was related to an injury sustained in her fall, but the location and persistence of her pain—in the middle of her back—was a red flag. Her

X ray showed a fracture in one of her vertebrae, and blood tests revealed elevation of blood proteins, consistent with a diagnosis of multiple myeloma, a bone marrow cancer. Obviously, her condition called for immediate medical intervention, and she went on to receive a course of chemotherapy. Her back pain improved when the cancer was diagnosed and appropriately treated. While Mary's case clearly falls into the small percentage of cases in which the pain is caused by a medical disorder, her condition calls attention to the importance of addressing pain that does not subside or pain that worsens over time.

### Rare Psychological Causes

Psychological or mental illness is a relatively rare cause of acute low back pain. Depending on individual characteristics, psychologic illnesses cause or exacerbate pain through a variety of mechanisms. For example, in schizophrenic patients, hallucinations are a rare but real cause of pain.

The psychiatric disorder commonly associated with low back pain is a **conversion reaction**: a mechanism for transforming anxiety or other emotions into a physical dysfunction. The symptoms lessen anxiety and symbolize the underlying conflict. Sufferers may benefit from their situation and may not be overly concerned about the physical problem. An abnormal body function, like back pain, is readily recognized and acceptable, but the perception is that psychological problems are not so easily accepted.

Someone with conversion reactions may have severe pain of a burning or cutting quality. The pain is excruciating in intensity and without any recognizable anatomic boundaries. On examination, they have a marked response to minimal pressure on palpation. Their areas of tenderness do not correspond to the tender points of fibromyalgia. Laboratory test results are normal, and in these patients, complaints are resistant to all forms of therapy. Unfortunately, even when the reason for the conversion reaction is evident, these patients may not improve.

Mark is a patient of mine with back pain related to a conversion reaction. He asked for a consultation with me about the need for surgery to relieve his back pain. He had an unfortunate history of work-related trauma. He was a building construction worker who had survived a back injury after falling from a two-story building. His back pain improved but he did not want to go up in buildings any more. He decided to work on the ground, paving roads. One day while leveling asphalt he was hit by a dump truck. He was hospitalized for back pain for a short period of time. He gradually recovered and was able to work again. He tried to look for other work but his educational background made construction his only option. To his misfortune, he was traumatized a third time when he was struck by a car while directing traffic around a highway paving project. This time Mark's back pain was unrelenting. The pain was constant, severe, and extensive in his back and legs. He was evaluated by other physicians with a variety of X ray techniques but only age-related changes could be seen. In desperation to help his problem, he was offered back surgery to remove the portion of his vertebral discs that were **bulging**. He was evaluated by me to advise him whether surgery would help his pain. After listening to his story, I became convinced that he was experiencing a conversion reaction. He was fearful that he would not survive his next accident and he did not want to be put in danger again. Vocational rehabilitation was the most effective therapy in Mark's circumstance. Only when he realized that he would not be placed in harm's way did his back pain improve.

On most days our back works perfectly well without any discomfort. On those days, we are able to sit at our computers, exercise at the gym, and enjoy lovemaking without a problem. Knowing how our back is put together goes a long way in trying to prevent back pain from happening.

## HOW YOUR BACK WORKS

After more than thirty years of caring for people with back pain, I've learned that taking the time to explain the anatomy and biomechanics of the lumbar spine goes a long way in helping people understand their situation and alleviate anxiety and fear.

Because most people have no idea of what caused their back problem in the first place, they often experience the same injuries again and again. On the other hand, I've seen people become so afraid of bringing on more pain, even with normal body motion, that they become stiff—like statues. They do not realize that their rigid posture does not protect them from pain but perpetuates it.

People who don't understand the cause of their pain often do not understand the prescribed treatments, and they don't follow through with self-care, including the specific exercises they are told to perform daily. So understanding how your back works will help you get rid of pain if you have it and prevent it if you are pain-free.

### The Lumbar Discs and Bony Joints

The lumbar spine is a beautifully engineered structure with two primary functions: movement and protection of the **spinal cord**. It is made up of bone, **discs**, ligaments, muscles, nerves, and blood vessels. The spine contains thirty-three vertebrae, each lined up one atop another and divided into five areas: **cervical** (neck), **thoracic** (chest), **lumbar** (low back), **sacral** (pelvis), and **coccyx** (tailbone).

- Cervical vertebrae facilitate motion in all directions.
- Thoracic vertebrae support the ribs and allow rotation of the body.
- Lumbar vertebrae support the upper part of the body and allow forward and backward motion.
- The **sacrum** acts as the anchor of the spine and fits between the pelvic bones.

When we look at the spine from the side, we can see that it is not straight, but curved. The neck and low back have forward-facing curves, while the chest and sacral spine have backward-facing curves (fig. 1.2). These curves allow room for the heart and lungs in the chest, while keeping the head centered over the lower body and the pelvis. This position is well balanced and strong.

Because each section of the spine serves a different function and motion, the vertebrae in each portion of the spine have specific shapes. The lumbar spine contains five vertebrae numbered one through five. You may hear a doctor refer to one of your vertebrae as L4, for example. This refers to the fourth lumbar vertebra. The assigned letters correspond to the section of the spine.

#### Facet Joints

Joints are formed where vertebrae meet at top and bottom. Each vertebra has four **facet joints**, two formed with each vertebra directly above and below, right and left. The vertical orientation allows for bending forward, the greatest degree of motion, and backward, a lesser degree of motion. The structure and orientation of the lumbar facet joints limit the twisting motions of the lumbar spine. The greatest rotation

**Cervical**

**Thoracic**

**Lumbar**

**Sacral and Coccygeal**

Figure 1.2. From the side you can see how the curves of your spine work to keep your body balanced so your head is directly over the center of gravity in your pelvis. Notice the balance between the forward curves (lordosis) of the neck and low back and the backward-facing curves (kyphosis) of the chest and pelvis.

of your spine occurs in the chest, the thoracic portion. The facet joints have cartilage on their surfaces, lining tissue (synovium) that makes joint fluid, and a joint covering, a capsule that keeps the joint fluid in and the bones together.

### The "His and Hers" Sacroiliac

The sacrum is a large triangular bone formed by five fused vertebrae wedged between the pelvic bones. The top of the sacrum is the first sacral vertebra, or S1. The sacroiliac joints are formed between the sacrum and the iliac bones. In this part of the spine, we can see male and female anatomical differences. In men, more of the sacrum is attached to the ilium, and in women, the sacroiliac joints widen during childbirth. These differences also play a role in the typical gait we associate with men and women. In men, the hip structure tends to be stable during normal walking movements; in women there is a natural sway of the hips. The sacrum contains the end of the spinal canal and, therefore, nerves.

The tailbone, as the coccyx is also known, consists of four tiny fused vertebrae located between the cheeks of the buttocks. This is well padded, which makes it difficult to fracture.

## Why You Are Taller in the Morning: Discs Are Cushions and Spacers

The **intervertebral** discs are the cushions between the vertebral bodies (bones) and make up about one-third of the entire height of the lumbar spine. The discs work like universal joints, allowing motion in a number of directions. If vertebral bodies were in direct contact with each other, range of motion would be severely limited.

The disc resembles an automobile tire with a strong balloon filled with a thick gel in the center, where the hub would be in a tire (fig. 1.3). The outer portion of the tire is the **annulus fibrosus**, layers of fiber that contract or expand, much like a Chinese finger trap. As we age, the restraining fibers break, and the ability to contain the gel at the center of the disc is compromised or weakened. If the gel moves beyond the boundary of the annulus fibrosus, we have an injury known as a herniated disc, often inaccurately called a slipped disc.

The gel portion of the disc can move forward or backward within the constraints of the "outer tire." The gel moves in opposition to the motion of the spine: forward motion of the spine moves the gel into the back portion of the disc; backward motion does the opposite. The gel can also move side to side. In addition to its ability to facilitate motion,

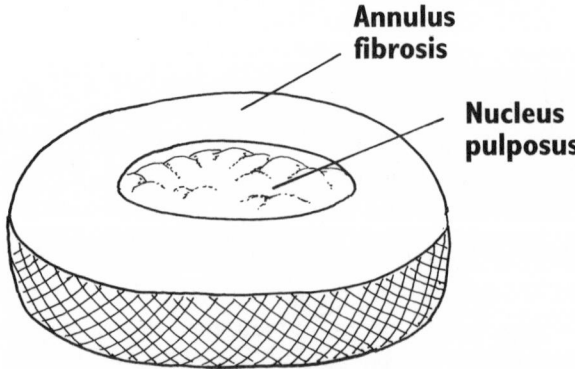

**Annulus fibrosis**

**Nucleus pulposus**

Figure 1.3.   The spinal disc looks much like an automobile tire, with a gel-like center surrounded by a fibrous outer circle.

the gel serves as a tremendous shock absorber. If the discs were structured without built-in shock absorbers, our bones would register the full impact of every step we take, and we would have a constant and awful headache.

A disc's cushioning ability depends upon how well the gel remains filled with water. At birth, 88 percent of the gel is water, but this changes as we age. It also changes during the course of the day. At night when there is no pressure on the discs, the gel swells, and we are taller in the morning. As we stand during our waking hours, the weight of the body compresses the discs, making them lose water, and by the end of the day, we are actually shorter. The fact that discs are "fatter" in the morning has some implications for the best time to exercise. As we grow older, the gel in the discs loses water and becomes more easily damaged by daily activities.

The discs not only allow motion between vertebrae, but also act as spacers between the bones. If you look at two vertebrae and a disc from the side (fig. 1.4), you will see a hole, or foramen, between the pedicles above and below the disc in front and the facet joint in back. This allows the nerves to exit the spine to supply other parts of the body. Any disease process that closes the hole has the potential to cause significant back and leg pain by pressing on the exiting nerves.

Figure 1.4. This side view of two vertebrae and a disc shows how the spinal bones fit together to protect the nerve root. The opening, called the neural foramen, allows the nerve roots to pass through the spine. Disc damage (herniation) or facet joint **degeneration** (bone spurs) may narrow the neural foramen, causing compression of the spinal nerve root and resulting in back or leg pain.

## Ligaments Are Like Rubber Bands

Ligaments are strong bands of tissue that act like a girdle or brace around the spine. Both front and back ligaments are closely attached to the outside surfaces of the bone and disc. This "outside packaging" helps keep the parts of the spine in the correct position. The posterior longitudinal ligament (PLL) covers the back of the vertebral bodies from your head to your pelvis and forms the front surface of the spinal canal. It narrows as it passes down the spine and is half its original width by the time it reaches the lumbar spine, and its ability to support discs is weakened. This is why the lumbar area is where disc injury is most likely to occur.

There are other spinal ligaments and all improve stability and restrain excessive movement of the spine. The ligaments act like strong, thick rubber bands, with some give but not too much. Their function is to lend support while limiting motion. The ligaments with more elastic fibers move farther than those without them. As part of the mechanism to accommodate childbirth, women have more elastic fibers than men. In both sexes, all these structures lose elasticity and become stiff with age, which is one reason we lose motion as the years accumulate.

## Back Muscles Are Not Our Strongest

Back muscles are among the weakest muscles for the kind of work they are called upon to do, but they play an essential role in the movement of the lumbar spine, as well as in maintaining normal posture (fig. 1.5). A number of muscles in the front of the abdomen and surrounding the spine also play a role in both balancing and moving the low back. The largest, but not necessarily the strongest, muscle runs from the base of the skull to the sacrum. This muscle pulls the spine backward and to

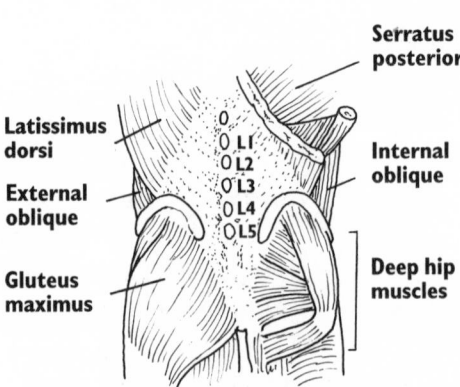

Figure 1.5.   Looking at the lumbar spine from the back, you can see the superficial low back muscles on the left and the deeper muscles on the right.

**Latissimus dorsi**

**External oblique**

**Gluteus maximus**

**Serratus posterior**

**Internal oblique**

**Deep hip muscles**

one side. Smaller muscles allow the spine to bend to the side and perform twisting motions. The psoas is a strong muscle that connects the low back with the thigh (fig. 1.6).

Although not officially part of the low back, muscles in the front and sides of the abdomen, the buttocks, the thighs, the **hamstrings**, and calves all play a role in balancing the spine. The abdominal muscles, including the rectus abdominis—the muscle that looks like two columns of rectangles on the front of body builders—have two major purposes. They bend the spine forward, and they also push the organs of the abdomen against the front of the spine, thereby lending it support. Muscles in the buttocks, thighs, and hamstrings need to be flexible to allow rotation around the hips. If these muscles are stiff, normal motion of the spine is limited, which may then result in low back pain.

All the muscles of your lower back are covered with **fascia**, a membrane that resembles plastic wrap. It surrounds individual muscles and

**Quadratus lumborum**

**Psoas**

Figure 1.6.　This view of the lumbar spine allows you to see how your muscles help the spine move. You can bend forward with the help of the psoas muscle and to the side with the quadratus lumborum.

connects them to neighboring muscles. A layer of fascia runs over a major portion of the lumbar spine, just below the skin. This "plastic wrap" enclosure improves the function of the contracting muscles, and while resilient, it does not contract as muscles do. Fascial tissue is supplied with nerves, and if it stretches or tears, with or without damage to the underlying muscle, it may cause pain.

### Nerves: Your Body's Pain Communication System

The role of the nervous system in low back pain is particularly complex because the nervous system itself is so amazing, far more complex than any computer software. However, basic knowledge of the anatomy of the nervous system is essential to understanding the specific pain patterns associated with back pain.

The spinal cord is the major nerve in the spinal canal, and it is constantly sending messages back and forth from the brain to various parts of the body. Moving your big toe, for example, starts with electrical signals that are relayed down the motor nerve column of your spinal cord and through the muscle in your lower leg that lifts your toe. Signals from sensory nerves in your big toe go back up the same nerve through a different sensory column in your spinal cord and report to your brain that the job has been accomplished. Your toe moved.

The spinal cord also has reflexive or involuntary functions, which are controlled by a single level in the spinal cord and do not require intervention from the brain. Let's say your big toe bumps into a rock. The sensory pain nerves send a signal to the sensory column in your spinal cord to report an injury. Your sensory nerve sends a signal to move to the motor nerve at the same level in your spinal cord. Then, through reflexive action, your foot quickly withdraws from pain.

Under normal conditions, you cannot measure the time between the bump and withdrawal because the entire sequence is faster than the split second it takes to mutter "ouch." This **reflex** requires that the sensory and motor nerves work together at a single level of the spinal cord. If a spinal nerve is compressed near the spinal canal, the reflex associated with that nerve may not work.

The spinal cord runs from the base of the brain to about the first lumbar vertebra. At that point, spinal nerves stretch through the sacrum to supply the legs. The brain, spinal cord, and spinal nerves are covered with the **dura**. This membrane contains the spinal fluid that bathes the brain, cord, and nerves.

The nerve root, as mentioned, passes through a hole in the vertebra—the foramen—and occupies a third of the available space. The rest of the space contains blood vessels, connective tissue, and the sensory nerve for the spine itself, the sinuvertebral nerve. Sensory and muscle functions are separated in the nerve root, and the sensory fibers are affected first when a nerve is compressed. This is why you feel pain before you lose strength. The L5 is the largest nerve root and is housed in the smallest lumbar foramen, so it is the most vulnerable to compression.

Nerve signals are interconnected with others and spread everywhere, making it hard to find the exact source of pain. Pain travels. Picture the nerves as the cables of a computer network that coordinate function and sensation (fig. 1.7). A single spinal nerve supplies the facet joint, the muscles and skin over the back, and the muscles, bone, and skin of the leg. When the nerve is irritated near the neural foramen, a signal is sent down the nerve reporting an injury. Any structure on that network,

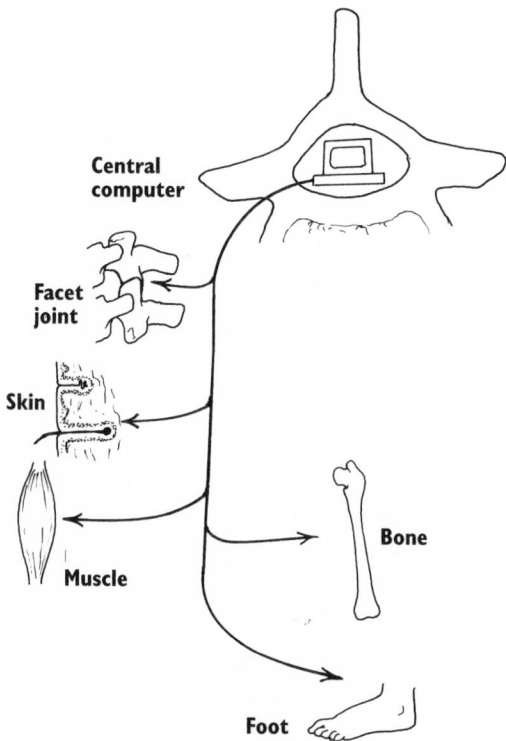

Figure 1.7. A spinal nerve as a computer network. An injury in one part of the system may affect the network at a distance from the main computer.

even though it is not damaged, may hurt in response to the injury at the level of the spine. An unpleasant sensation experienced away from the original location of injury is called referred pain. People who suffer from back pain and related symptoms are often surprised that their spine is actually the source of numbness in their foot, for example.

## PAIN IS DIFFERENT IN MEN AND WOMEN

The International Association for the Study of Pain defines pain as "an unpleasant sensory and emotional experience which we primarily associate with tissue damage or describe in terms of such damage, or both." The definition of pain has two parts. One part deals with tissue damage or the threat of damage, but to experience pain one must have an emotional response to that injury. Mental stress may elicit an emotional response that is experienced as pain. Pain may be generated in the arms, legs, or back but is experienced in the brain. Pain has become an ever increasingly complicated biologic process produced by multiple interactions. These interactions involve your **genes**, your sex hormones, and the chemicals your nerves manufacture to transmit signals to the brain. Women have a greater risk for the development of chronic pain. This is partly due to estrogen, the female hormone. For example, decreased function of a specific enzyme results in the overproduction of signal chemicals that result in a more painful condition. Estrogen facilitates the decreased function of that enzyme causing increased stimulation of the pain pathway. These differences could explain, in part, the different responses of men and woman to pain therapies prescribed for back disorders.

## HOW YOUR PAIN THRESHOLD FLUCTUATES

If you are under increasing levels of stress, you will be more sensitive to pain. Your pain threshold will be lower. Let's say you stub your big toe with the same force on a Monday morning and a Friday afternoon. On Monday you are rested after an enjoyable weekend. You had a wonderful time and feel well. Your stubbed toe does not hurt very much at all. On Friday, you are exhausted from all the decisions you made during the week. The service people have not come to fix the fax machine, two of the staff are out with the flu, and the deadline for the project is next week. Stress is your middle name. You stub your toe on your desk and you think your foot is going to fall off. The pain is intense. The same amount of injury is felt with a different intensity of pain.

Pain signals to the brain and their perception as pain can be modified by a number of mechanisms. **Acupuncture**, massage, transcutaneous electrical nerve stimulation (TENS), or surface magnets held by Velcro wraps are a few examples of therapies that put sensations into the nervous system to modify signals that are different than the slow pain signals. We'll get to these later in the book.

Another mechanism that blocks pain is the body's production of its own pain relievers, **endorphins**. These chemicals attach to **opioid** receptors in the nerve pathways that block the transmission of pain signals. The release of these endorphins can be accomplished in a number of ways, such as regular exercise. A positive outlook and a reduction of stress can also release endorphins. The belief that a good outcome will be the result of an interaction can have beneficial effects on the healing process, partly mediated through the release of endorphins.

---

### DR. B'S PRESCRIPTION SUMMARY

- Ninety percent of back pain is mechanical in origin.
- Mechanical back pain is secondary to overuse or aging.
- Red flags of fever, night pain, prolonged morning stiffness, bone pain, or cramps identify systemic illnesses that are causing back pain.
- Your lumbar spine has five vertebrae (L1–L5) and discs supported by ligaments and muscles.
- Your spinal cord is the communications center for transmitting pain impulses and messages between your body and brain.
- Pain travels; injury in one structure, such as a joint, can cause pain in another structure, such as a muscle connected on the same nerve network.
- Your perception of pain can vary for many reasons, including your level of stress.
- Men and women have different risks for the development of chronic pain related to genetics and sex hormones.
- When your back is weak you are at more risk for injury. The major muscle supporting your lower back is among the weakest in your body.

---

# Chapter 2

# Working with Your Doctor

YOUR DOCTOR NEEDS a complete picture of you and your back pain before he or she can get to the bottom of the problem. During the telling of your story and a physical examination, any one fact may be the clue that solves the puzzle of your back pain. In fact, most diagnoses are established during the history portion of the examination. The rest of the process identifies the correct diagnosis from the variety of possibilities developed by your description of your back pain.

Your age and gender, naturally, are important to a correct diagnosis. For example, more herniated discs occur between the ages of twenty-five and forty-five. Conversely, approximately 80 percent of people with cancer of the spine are fifty or older. Men have back pain more frequently than women, some of which may be explained by occupational exposure to more physically strenuous work. Certain disorders occur exclusively or predominantly in women, such as back pain during pregnancy and **osteoporosis**. (Men are at risk for this thinning of the bones, too, but the risk is greater for postmenopausal women.)

The history you provide is the most important part of the diagnostic process. The more complete the information, the greater its value. Every subsequent step is used to confirm the ideas and even hunches developed during the medical history. The first part of your history, the chief complaint, is your description of what brought you to the doctor. In most circumstances, the chief complaint is "I have a pain in my back." Another frequent chief complaint is "I have a pain in my back that runs down my leg to my foot." Your description guides the doctor's questions.

Telling your story allows you to describe those events that you believe are most important in explaining the evolution of your back pain. Your doctor may or may not ask questions as you progress with your narrative. A physician may interrupt to ask a question if a particular point is essential to differentiate between diagnostic possibilities. For example, you may be asked: "Did the pain that ran down your leg go to your big toe or small toe?"

Help yourself and your doctor by gathering your thoughts about your back pain and organizing the description of your symptoms and questions you want to ask. Perhaps you can store the information in your head, but writing it down may be more useful. By carefully thinking about your back pain, you will have organized information necessary to start the diagnostic process. Also, bring a list of your medicines—or the actual medicines—with you and the names and addresses of your other health care providers.

## QUESTIONS TO HELP YOU FIND THE CAUSE

### When Did the Pain Begin?

Acute onset of back pain is most closely associated with a specific episode of trauma to the spine, such as lifting a heavy bag of groceries from the back seat of your car. In contrast, systemic illnesses cause pain that is gradual in onset. People with inflammatory arthritis of the spine (**spondyloarthropathy**) may have had back stiffness and pain for six months or longer when first evaluated for their spine symptoms.

### How Long Does It Last and How Often Does It Occur?

The initial episodes of mechanical low back pain resolve over days. With successive episodes, the duration of pain increases to a week and then a month; episodes may be intermittent over time. The frequency of pain follows environmental exposure, such as shoveling snow in winter or several hours of weeding the garden in the summer.

For medical low back pain, the important characteristic is duration, not frequency. As opposed to the short duration of mechanical low back pain, medical low back pain is more persistent. It may last for months, with minimal variation in discomfort.

### Where Is It Located and Where Else Do You Feel It?

Most low back pain is localized between the lower rib and buttocks, where the spinal curve (**lordosis**) is greatest. Frequently, the pain starts to one side of the spine and quickly spreads across the low back.

The fleshy part of the back is more commonly affected than the bones themselves. Occasionally pain will be present on both sides of the spine, near the "dimples" just above the buttocks, over the sacroiliac joints. Sometimes the location and radiation of pain is very difficult to describe because it is referred pain, that is, it comes from somewhere else (see chapter 1). Pain can move side to side, or up and down the leg. However, the most important facts are where the pain first started and how far the pain has spread.

## What Makes It Feel Worse or Better?

Mechanical low back pain disorders improve with rest and worsen with certain activities. Muscle injuries are aggravated with stretching and are relieved when the muscle is at rest and therefore shortened in length. This resting position allows healing to take place. For example, a thirty-two-year-old man who picked up a heavy box of papers experienced immediate onset of right-sided low back pain. His pain increased with any movement of his spine forward (flexed) or to the left side. These motions stretched the injured muscles on the right side of his spine, thereby intensifying the pain. He was most comfortable when resting in bed or standing with a tilt to the right side.

Anything that increases pressure on discs will also increase compression of spinal nerves. If you have a herniated disc, you have increased pain with sitting, sneezing, coughing, or having a bowel movement. Disc pressure is reduced when you are standing up.

If you have more back pain standing, then you could have arthritis of the back joints. You probably have less pain when you sit. When leg pain occurs with standing, **spinal stenosis** is the most common diagnosis. Walking for a distance may be associated with leg pain. If you sit down or rest against a structure with your spine bent forward, your leg pain decreases.

Sarah is a seventy-two-year-old woman who was able to stand and walk with little discomfort whose pain was worse when she was sitting or lying in bed. She was frustrated because she was about to take a trip and was worried about sitting on the plane for an extended time. Why was she frustrated? She was given a diagnosis of spinal stenosis, or so her MRI scan reported. However, therapy for that problem had not helped. She had been to other doctors who read her report but did not listen to her complaints. Despite the findings in her spine, the cause of her problem was tension in her hamstring muscles. A gentle stretching exercise program and the addition of a muscle relaxant improved her condition. Her therapy treated her problem not the finding on her MRI report.

Alleviating and aggravating factors for medical low back pain are more complicated. Inflammatory arthritis can hurt more when you are not moving and hurt less with walking, bending, and stretching. Others with medical low back pain have severe low back pain unless they stay motionless. They may also have other signs of a serious illness such as fever, chills, or weight loss (remember those red flags).

### What Time of Day or Night Does It Occur?

Systemic disorders, like inflammatory arthritis, are most symptomatic during sleep or in the early morning while getting out of bed. Stiffness and pain are improved with normal movement as the day progresses. Conversely, people with tumors of the spine have increased pain when lying flat in bed. They usually sit in a chair to sleep, or they may walk around to relieve their pain.

Mechanical disorders become more symptomatic with use, and the greatest pain occurs at the end of the day.

### What Is the Quality and Intensity?

A wide variety of terms are used to describe pain. Skin disorders cause local burning pain on the surface of the body. Disorders of the bones, joints, muscles, and ligaments cause a deep, dull ache that is most intense over the involved site. A cramping pain is associated with reflex contraction of an injured muscle or from a muscle chronically contracted to protect an injured portion of the lumbar spine, like a facet joint.

Pain from nerve compression (radicular pain) has a sharp, shooting, burning quality that follows the distribution of the compressed nerve. This kind of pain is associated with **sciatica**, compression of the sciatic nerve. Other forms of nerve pain occur with direct trauma to the nerve or secondary to changes in the metabolism of the nerve, a situation associated with diabetes. This form of pain has a tingling and crushing component that is unaffected by physical position of the body but is intensified by touching of the skin supplied by the nerve. The severity of the pain may continue even after the stimulus is gone.

Kidney stones cause a recurrent gripping pain that rises quickly to its greatest intensity in twenty to thirty seconds, lasts one to two minutes, and then quickly resolves. Throbbing pain is associated with disorders of blood vessels. A tearing sensation is a potential sign of blood vessel injury that may cause loss of blood flow to structures in the lower extremities.

### Who Else in Your Family Has It?

Most disorders of the lumbar spine are not genetic. However, disc herniations and sciatica occurring in many family members suggests a relationship between your back and leg pain and family characteristics. The group of conditions known as inflammatory arthritis of the spine (spondyloarthropathies) has a genetic predisposition and a test could determine if you are at risk. Therefore, mention these disorders to your doctor as part of your family history.

### How Does Your Work or Lifestyle Affect It?

Your profession can determine your risk for developing low back pain. Other risk factors aside, heavy lifting and carrying on the job add to the risk for developing mechanical low back pain. Onset of pain while at work has potential implications for qualifying for worker's compensation. Be sure to tell your doctor if you see a relationship between your job and your back pain. If you sit all day at a computer, you may develop low back pain, and there's been lots of talk lately about **ergonomics**, posture chairs, and mouse pads. (See my Back School FAQ for information about chairs.)

Smoking tobacco and drinking alcohol are implicated in osteoporosis; they weaken the bones in your spine. (Alcohol may also limit the use of certain medications used to control pain and **inflammation**.) Think about the way your back pain affects activities and relationships with the important people in your life. Perhaps you are unable to participate in your basketball or bowling league or swing dancing. Back pain often has a detrimental effect on sexual relationships. When any simple motion increases your pain it is difficult to enjoy sex. Discuss these social and personal difficulties honestly with your physician so he or she can help you.

### Past and Present Medical History

Your medical history necessarily deals with past and current illnesses. For example, a history of cancer may have great significance in the onset of new back pain. A previous injury, such as slipping and falling on ice, may be the initiating event in the development of a herniated disc. A history of diabetes increases the risk for developing nerve irritation (neuropathy) that causes back and leg pain. Psoriasis and inflammatory bowel disease are associated with inflammatory arthritis of the spine. Eye inflammation may also be linked with back disorders. Illnesses such as hypertension may limit the use of certain medications because of side effects. Environmental or drug allergies should be mentioned as well.

## THE PHYSICAL EXAMINATION

Once your pain story and medical, social, and family histories have been obtained, you will move on to the second part of the diagnostic process—the physical examination of your lower back. Physicians each have their own methods for this examination, but here's what I look for.

### Lumbar Spine Examination

Your doctor will examine your spine while you are standing, sitting, and lying on your stomach to discover any abnormalities. Curvature of the spine (**scoliosis**) is associated with elevation of either shoulder and is best discovered when standing (fig. 2.1). Tilting the pelvis will show inequality in the length of the legs. From the side, it is easy to note a forward position of the head with a mound at attachment of the neck to the chest, which is known as a dowager's hump, or increased backward curve of the spine, **kyphosis** (fig. 2.2). Characteristics of poor posture are also best seen from the side. For example, if you have a protruding abdomen, it's a sign of weak abdominal muscles and you will have an increased forward lumbar curve, or hyperlordosis.

Figure 2.1.    Scoliosis has curved this spine to the right in the thoracic region and to the left in the low back. Notice the left shoulder is higher than the right shoulder. When bending forward, the left shoulder blade will be more prominent than the right. This structural abnormality affects young girls and is most effectively treated when identified early.

Figure 2.2. Kyphosis, a prominent bump between the shoulder blades, pushes the head forward.

Your doctor will touch your back with varying degrees of pressure to detect increased muscle contraction or spasm. Back muscles at rest can be compressed with gentle pressure because they are soft and moveable. Muscles in spasm are tense and firm to the touch and may be tender with direct palpation. More commonly, moving the tense muscle increases pain.

Both sides of your spine will be compressed to examine for symmetry of muscle contraction. In the resting upright position, spasm on one side of the lumbar spine may be detected while the other side of the spine is normal. This asymmetry of muscle contraction helps identify the location of the original injury, most often to muscle or fascia.

### Range of Motion and Rhythm

Tests for range of motion can tell us a great deal. For example, if you have increased back pain when you bend backward you may have arthritis of the facet joints (fig. 2.3). Thigh pain may also be an indication of abnormalities in organs located in the back of the abdomen. You will be asked

Figure 2.3. Bending the lumbar spine backward is called extension. Bending forward is called flexion.

to bend forward from a standing position, bend to both sides, bend backward, and rotate your hips. (The total range of motion of the spine is not always as important as the natural rhythm of motion.)

An injured lumbar spine will have limited normal motion because the muscles will tighten to protect it. The lumbar spine will not have the normal curve in the standing position, nor will the lumbar curve reverse. Forward movement of the spine is severely limited. If injury to the spine is unilateral, the spine is tilted to the side of the shortened muscles in spasm. There may also be limited ability to bend the knees (**flexion**), which results from tightness of the buttocks and hamstring muscles in the back of the thigh.

When you bend and return to an upright position, the motion can reveal information about the injured structures causing pain. Normally, the hips are rotated first, and the lower spine goes from being bent forward to bent backward. When an injury affects the spine, the spine is bent backward first, and bending the knees and rotating the hips establish the upright posture (fig. 2.4).

Bending to one side stretches the muscles on the opposite side of your spine and compresses spinal joints on the same side as the motion. Pain just to the side of the midline on the same side as the motion suggests irritation of the facet joint at that level of the spine. Pain from compression of the facet joint may radiate down the leg to the foot. A stretching sensation with pain on the side opposite the motion suggests a muscle injury with spasm (fig. 2.5).

### Testing Muscles and Reflexes

When you are lying flat on your back on the examining table, your doctor may raise your leg up in the air. This maneuver puts a strain on your sciatic nerve (fig. 2.6), so if there is nerve compression, your leg pain will get worse with this test. If the pain is not in your leg, but in your lower back or buttock, this suggests a problem in joints or muscles without nerve irritation. The doctor may bend your knee and rotate your leg from side to side while you lie on your side. This movement tests the integrity of your hip, and arthritis in the hip causes pain in the groin and buttock. Also, patients with piriformis **syndrome** (see chapter 5) have pain in the buttock and down the thigh toward the calf when moving the bent leg toward the center of the body.

The sensory and reflex examination is done while you are seated with your legs dangling. The doctor will touch both your legs with a pin

**Normal**

**A**

**B**

Figure 2.4. Normally, bending backward and simultaneously rotating your hips (A) is a fluid and effortless motion. When your back is in pain, however, the motion is abnormal (B) and relies on rotating your hips and bending your knees. This motion is hesitant and fatiguing.

or a tuning fork and ask if you can tell the difference in sensation. This helps pinpoint which nerve is causing numbness. Numbness between the legs is associated with disorders of the lower sacral nerve roots. Hitting your knee and the back of your ankle with a rubber hammer is another test of reflexes. An absence of knee reflex, for example, corresponds to an abnormality of the L4 nerve root.

Toe raises repeated ten times determine a difference in strength in the calf muscles. Walking on your heels tests the stamina of your shin muscles and big toe. A deep knee bend tests the strength of all your lower extremity muscles (fig. 2.7).

Figure 2.5. When pain is on the same side (A) as the direction of movement, it is associated with bone pain from facet joint disease. Pain on the opposite side as the direction of movement (B) is associated with a muscle injury.

Figure 2.6.    By raising your leg straight, you stretch the sciatic nerve. In this position, pain that radiates below your knee may indicate a herniated disc.

**A**

**B**

**Toe raise**

**Flex**

**C**

**Squat**

Figure 2.7.    These three tests measure the strength of the calf (A), shin (B), and thigh (C).

## Other Tests

A targeted musculoskeletal examination will concentrate on the lumbar spine and may not evaluate other portions of the skeletal system. However, if you have joint pain in other areas, then it is appropriate to examine all the joints.

In addition to the joints, other organ systems may be evaluated if the medical history has identified specific disorders such as heart failure or gastrointestinal ulcers. A rectal examination may be necessary if loss of bowel control has occurred along with back pain. This examination is also appropriate for determining the status of the prostate gland in a man with persistent back pain.

The history and physical examination are often all we need to determine the likely cause of a back attack and additional tests are unnecessary before starting therapy. However, X ray and blood tests potentially corroborate the initial impression gained through the medical evaluation. (The next chapter outlines what these tests can and cannot do.)

## DOCTORS AND HEALTH CARE PROFESSIONALS
## WHO TREAT LOW BACK PAIN

I am a rheumatologist. Rheumatology is a subspecialty of internal medicine dealing with the treatment of patients with arthritis or any disorders in the bones, joints, or muscles. We prescribe **nonsteroidal anti-inflammatory** drugs (NSAIDs—aspirin-like drugs), muscle relaxants, and physical therapy. To find a rheumatologist in your community, either an M.D. or D.O., check with your local Arthritis Foundation or the American College of Rheumatology.

A number of other physicians and health care professionals take care of back pain patients.

- Internist/Family practitioner: An allopathic (M.D.) or osteopathic (D.O.) physician who is a primary care professional offering general health care needs, including general back therapy.
- Neurologist: M.D. or D.O. specializing in the diagnosis and treatment of nerve disorders; this doctor has special skills in the diagnosis of nerve abnormalities, including electrodiagnostic tests.
- Physiatrist: M.D. or D.O. specializing in rehabilitation of the musculoskeletal and nervous systems, who offers special skills in electrodiagnostic tests, exercise methods, and body supports.
- Orthopedic surgeon: M.D. or D.O. who is a specialist in the surgery of the skeletal system, including the spine.
- Neurosurgeon: M.D. or D.O. specializing in the surgery of the nervous system, including the spine.

- Anesthesiologist/Pain management practitioner: M.D. or D.O. specializing in diagnosis and treatment of pain, who offers special skills in injections of painful areas.
- Interventional radiologist: M.D. or D.O. specializing in the use of radiographic techniques to place injections.
- Physical therapist: P.T., R.P.T. (registered), or M.P.T. (master's) specializing in the use of exercise and physical methods to relieve pain and restore function.
- Chiropractor: D.C. (doctor of chiropractic) who uses physical adjustments and mobilization to treat spinal disorders.
- Acupuncturist: A health professional who places needles at various points of the body to unblock energy to treat spinal disorders.
- Massage therapist: L.M.T. (licensed massage therapist) who uses therapeutic muscle massage to improve musculoskeletal disorders.

Chose your health care provider depending on your specific back problem, but always start with your primary care physician or rheumatologist. See a surgeon if you have muscle weakness or have failed medical therapy.

---

### DR. B'S PRESCRIPTION SUMMARY

- Be prepared. Knowing the characteristics of your back pain will make the time with your health care provider more efficient.
- The most important part of the back evaluation is your own complete medical and lifestyle history.
- The specific character of back pain helps define its source.
- The physical examination identifies abnormalities of normal movement, sensation, muscle strength, and reflexes.
- Most back evaluations do not require additional X ray or blood tests.
- Your primary care physician or rheumatologist can start your back evaluation and offer appropriate referrals if additional therapy is needed.

Chapter 3

# What Diagnostic Tests Can—
# and Cannot—Tell You

WHEN NEW PATIENTS come to my office, I always pick up their charts from the plastic holder on the door to the examining room. This plastic holder may also contain a large envelope of **X rays** or **magnetic resonance imaging** (MRI) studies of the lumbar spine. I peruse the chart to familiarize myself with the patient I'm about to meet, but I do not open the large folder and study the test results.

After introducing myself, I ask new patients to tell me the reason they scheduled an appointment. They usually respond by mentioning their back pain; then they ask if I have reviewed the X rays and MRI results they brought. Invariably, I see their disappointment when I tell them I have not looked at these tests. This disappointment is understandable, because they have gone to the trouble of supplying the information and believe they are being "good patients." However, there is a method to what may seem like madness. Patients eventually understand my thinking when I explain why I like to hear about their problems and examine them first before reviewing their X rays or MRI results.

Diagnostic "pictures" have importance only in the context of your current clinical complaints. Any number of abnormalities may appear on the X rays or MRI, but these results may be of little consequence in explaining and treating the problem that prompted a visit to a new doctor.

I repeat this scenario with patients again and again, and it serves to shed light on both the advantages and disadvantages of rapid advancements in medical technology. We now have the ability to look inside the human body and obtain highly detailed images without exposing people to radiation. The MRI scanner uses large magnets and radio waves and presents visual images of the structures in the spine that were difficult to see with older, radiation-based technology. The **computed axial tomography** scan (CT) uses X rays (radiation) to identify structures in and around the spine. We can put multiple CT pictures together to achieve a three-dimensional view of the spine.

## PICTURES MAY NOT TELL THE WHOLE STORY

Most of us are impressed by what these imaging machines can do, and no question, they represent important progress in medicine. But just because we can see the spine in better ways than ever before does not mean that we have significantly increased our understanding of what causes back pain.

Our enthusiasm for medical technology must be tempered by recognizing that changes or deviations from what we define as "normal" are not necessarily associated with a specific complaint. In fact, most changes from normal are asymptomatic. Patients may tell me that an MRI scan has documented bulging discs at two or three levels. They are concerned that their bulging discs must be the source of their pain. However, a number of X ray studies have discovered bulging discs at multiple levels of the spine in people without any back pain.

The lack of correlation between clinical symptoms and X ray findings is characteristic of the most common causes of low back pain, which are mechanical disorders of the lumbar spine. Based on autopsy findings, by age fifty up to 95 percent of adults show evidence of changes in the spine due to aging, including disc space narrowing. In X ray studies of people fifty or older, 87 percent have demonstrated changes in the intervertebral discs, due again, to aging.

In 1984, the medical journal *Spine* reported research findings that remain important in our understanding that the reason for pain may not be related to what we can see on a picture. This study compared X ray test results of 238 patients with back pain and 66 without pain. In terms of the prevalence of disc degeneration, researchers could detect no difference between the two groups.

MRI scans are no better at identifying patients with back pain than plain X rays. In 1989, a study reported on lumbar spine MRI findings in 67 asymptomatic subjects. Radiologists found 31 percent with identifiable abnormalities that are associated with pain. The interesting finding, of course, is all those individuals had no back pain. MRI scans can identify anatomic alterations from normal but they do not identify those who are in pain. Also, MRI scans do not predict who will develop pain. A follow-up MRI study was completed on 50 of those 67 people who were subjects in 1989. In 1996, the individuals with the greatest degree of anatomic abnormality in prior study were not the people who had the greatest amount of back pain. This study tells us that changes on MRI scan only become important when they correlate with your clinical complaints.

However, keep in mind that while many changes in the spine detectable through X ray testing do not cause pain, other abnormalities have significant consequences and require further evaluation. What remains important is knowing when to get X ray testing and what such testing says about the health of the spine. Most people with back pain get better without any of these tests.

## CONVENTIONAL X RAYS

Generally, you will not require X rays of the lumbar spine during the early stages of your back attack except when there are signs of a medical cause of back pain. These are the red flags mentioned earlier and include fever, weight loss, or history of cancer. In most circumstances, X rays are not required unless you've been in pain for six to eight weeks.

I order X rays of the lumbar spine if I am concerned about medical disorders of the spine, including arthritis that affects the facet joints. I do not order X rays if a soft tissue problem such as muscle **strain** is causing pain. If pain has been present for more than six to eight weeks, or for individuals over age fifty with persistent pain, then X ray testing is usually called for.

Generally, you will be positioned on your back and on your side for an initial X ray study. Oblique (on an incline) views, required less frequently, are taken with the X ray tube at a forty-five-degree slant to your body. If there is a concern about the stability of your spine, you may have flexion (bending forward) and **extension** (bending backward) views of the lumbar spine. In your day-to-day activities, these bending motions place forces on the spine that may cause shifting of the vertebrae if they are not fully anchored by the facet joints (**spondylolisthesis**). A routine view of the pelvis, which images the sacroiliac and hip joints, is taken while you are flat on the X ray table.

Plain X rays are excellent at photographing the spatial arrangement of the vertebrae (fig. 3.1), and they show the distance between vertebrae, which indicates the health of the corresponding disc. These pictures also detect changes in bony architecture that may be altered by the presence of prostate or breast cancer or osteoporosis. X rays use ionizing radiation to generate images. Minimizing exposure to ionizing radiation is important to limit the risk for developing cancer.

Modern X ray testing equipment does the same work as older machinery but minimizes exposure to radiation while remaining the least expensive radiographic technique. Digital X ray is the new state-of-the-art lower radiation technique that allows for highlighting abnormalities that would have not been recognized by older X ray methods. The cost of lumbar spine series ranges from $180 to $300.

Figure 3.1. From the front, this plain X ray of a lumbar spine (A) reveals no abnormalities. From the side, however (B), we can see a mild narrowing of the last vertebral body and the sacrum (black arrow). This narrowing indicates disc degeneration.

MRI is the most recently developed diagnostic imaging technique for medical conditions such as low back pain. Through the use of radio waves and magnets, with some strengths greater than the magnetic field around the earth, this noninvasive technique images the component parts of the lumbar spine from a number of directions. The anatomy of the intervertebral disc, spinal nerves, ligaments, facet joints, and adjacent muscles are visualized (fig. 3.2), and intervertebral disc herniations are easily identified.

Contrast dye (**gadolinium**) may be injected into a vein if additional information is needed to determine the amount of blood flow to a specific area of the spine. Increased blood flow occurs in areas where scarring from previous back surgeries or tumors is present. The use of gadolinium for MR scanning is usually unassociated with any side effects. However, you should be cautious if you have severe kidney failure. You may be at risk of developing a generalized scarring process that can affect the skin and internal organs.

### Open versus Closed

Many of my patients ask questions about the type of scanner that should be used to get their MRI images. They have heard of closed and open machines and wonder which is best. In a closed machine, you are on your back and placed in a confining, hollow tube. The tube is open on both ends. The top of the tube is two to three inches from your face. Depending on the number of views needed, the test lasts between twenty and sixty minutes, and the machine makes a ticking sound during the scans.

For those with claustrophobia, an open MRI is available. The open machines come in various forms but usually consist of round magnets supported by four columns. The scanner is open on all sides. The concern about open scanners is that the images are less sharp than those produced by the closed "tube" version. Open scanner images are improving on a regular basis, but will not be able to match pictures generated by closed machines.

Sedation prior to a closed scan is effective to calm claustrophobic patients. Oral forms of therapy work just as fast as injectable forms. Bringing along a companion can be helpful in calming you while in the machine. I inform patients that they will be saving time in getting at the cause of their problem by getting a closed MRI scan.

Figure 3.2.   With an MRI view from the side of this lumbar spine
(A) we can see that there is a disc herniation at the L5-S interspace
(white arrow). A cross-sectional view (B) identifies the disc herniation on the left side (white arrow).

The MRI is a painless procedure, but if you are experiencing back pain you may be uncomfortable lying still on your back with your legs straight for the length of time needed to complete the examination. MRI involves no exposure to radiation, but it is not used if you have metal clips with magnetic properties in your body from surgery. There is a risk that the clips will move under the influence of the magnet. The MRI machine will also short-circuit a pacemaker.

A new development in MRI technology is the open standing machine. You are able to sit or stand in this MRI scanner. The opportunity to sit or stand may be important if your pain is generated with standing or sitting. Most MRI scans are taken with you lying on your back. The supine MRI scan may explain, in part, why there is a lack of correlation between clinical symptoms and MRI pictures. The abnormality that causes pain may be seen only when you are standing: the position that causes your pain. The open standing MRI scanner is not as available as usual MRI machines. You will need to ask you doctor if the standing study is appropriate for you and if that scanner is available in your community.

The cost of an MRI ranges from approximately $1,300 to $2,600, and the higher figure is associated with the cost of two MRIs, one with and one without contrast. MRI scanners are available in most communities with a local hospital.

I can offer a personal perspective on this test because I had one myself. I was one of the subjects in the 1989 study I mentioned earlier in this chapter. The top of the tube was about two inches from my face, which is why those with claustrophobia have a difficult time with this test. I was told to remain still while the scans were completed. I frequently gazed toward my feet to assure myself that escape from the machine was possible. I was very glad to get out of the tube once the scans were over. Because of this experience, I am able to sympathize with my back pain patients who must undergo this test while they experience back discomfort. I promised myself that I would not send my patients for MRI testing unless the information was essential to their care.

MRIs are appropriate for those who have red flags for medical disorders and for those with sciatica (pain radiating from the back to the leg) who are considering **epidural** corticosteroid injections (see chapter 9) or lumbar spine surgery (see chapter 12). Bone abnormalities are better visualized by another radiographic technique.

The MRI scan is the most sensitive test for those who need radiographic evaluation to identify the location of the disc herniation and nerve compression. X rays may be entirely normal in individuals with a herniated disc, but MRI scans identify the location of disc herniations including the migration of extruded disc fragments. A CT scan can identify disc herniations in individuals who have metal in their bodies and are therefore unable to undergo MRI testing, but the CT does not offer the general overview of the spine that is obtained with the MRI machine.

MRI scans do not predict the development of pain in the lumbar spine. In a medical study, fifty people without back pain underwent MRI scans of the lumbar spine. Seven years later, they were asked whether they had developed back pain. People who developed low back pain had no greater abnormal changes on their MRI scans than those who remained pain-free. Repeat MRI scans on this group did not show any consistent pattern of disc changes. Some had improved while others had worsened on their scans. There was no correlation with those who felt better or worse.

## COMPUTED AXIAL TOMOGRAPHY (CT)

CT scans, sometimes called CAT scans, create cross-sectional (axial) images of the bony structure of the lumbar spine (fig. 3.3). With a computer, the images can be reformatted to form a three-dimensional model of the spine. CT scans also assess soft tissues including discs, ligaments, nerve roots, and fat. CT technology is appropriate for people with pacemakers, metal clips, or claustrophobia, who are therefore unable to have an MRI scan.

CT scans are taken while you lie flat on your back in the center of an open circular overhead structure that supports the scanning machine (gantry). This test does not cause pain except for the discomfort of lying still for twenty to forty minutes. Radiation exposure is three to five **rads**, with the greater exposure associated with higher-resolution scans. The cost ranges from $800 to $2,000, if a **myelogram** is required.

CT findings corroborate clinical impressions, but as with MRI results, abnormalities not associated with symptoms may be present in as many as 3o percent of people without pain. I order CT scans to reveal bony abnormalities occurring with central and lateral spinal stenosis (compression of spinal nerves), facet joint arthritis, fractures, and metastatic bone disease. CT is my second choice of image testing

Figure 3.3. A cross-sectional view with a CT scan reveals arthritis in both facet joints (arrows).

for identifying a herniated disc and by necessity is the first option for those with a pacemaker or claustrophobia.

Radiation exposure from CT scans is an increasing concern. CT studies of the abdomen and pelvis are associated with an increased risk of developing cancer. The amount of radiation for a lumbar spine study can be substantial. The increased risk of developing cancer is related to the duration of ionizing radiation exposure. Younger individuals are at greater risk than those who have CT scans later in life. The take home message is that you should have a CT scan if it is the only test that can diagnose your problem.

## MYELOGRAPHY

Before the advent of MRI technology, the myelogram was the "gold standard" for X ray evaluation of the lumbar spine. The myelogram fell out of favor for a number of reasons, one of which is the need to inject a contrast dye into the spinal canal, thereby making it an invasive test. A headache may develop after the exam and in rare circumstances a seizure can be caused by the dye. Despite its limitations, the myelogram allows you to stand or bend while the films are exposed. The ability to test in a "functional" position is particularly helpful for diagnosing spinal stenosis. Myelography is also an important radiographic technique for spinal surgery patients with metal rods because the presence of metal spoils the ability of MRI or CT scans to visualize the spine.

Like MRI and CT, myelography is associated with anatomical abnormalities without pain. Just like the other tests, clinical judgment is important in evaluating the myelogram. I rarely order a myelogram or CT-myelogram and only use the test for patients considering surgery for spinal stenosis and who want to know the extent of the bone removal required to improve their condition.

Because the dye eventually becomes diluted, a myelogram must be completed in twenty to thirty minutes. However, because of the spinal puncture, you must sit for two hours and then lie down for two hours. Resting in these positions diminishes the risk of headaches. X ray exposure is six to seven rads, and the cost is approximately $1,200.

## BONE SCAN

Bone scan (**radionuclide** imaging) is a useful test to detect bone abnormalities or fractures. The bone scan involves an injection of a small amount of a radioactive material into your vein. A few hours following the injection, the scanning portion of the test begins. You are flat on your stomach for up to sixty minutes while the lumbar spine is scanned. Areas of the skeleton that are reacting to an injury (fracture or inflammation) show up as a dark or "hot" spot on the scan. Most bone cells in the skeleton are in a dormant state maintaining bone structure. The increased activity on the scan results from the increased absorption of the radioactive material by the bone cells trying to heal the injury. The presence of the "hot" spot does not indicate a specific diagnosis, because tumors, infections, fractures, and arthritis all cause dark spots on the scans. Additional radiographic evaluation or blood testing is needed to reach a specific diagnosis.

I order bone scans when I am concerned about the possibility of bone fractures in the spine. Some fractures are very small and are not seen by plain X rays. Bone scans are able to identify the location of these fractures regardless of the cause.

A bone scan is painless except for the discomfort associated with being flat for a period of time, which may increase your back pain. The radiation exposure is small, 0.15 rad, and the cost is approximately $600.

## DISCOGRAPHY

I do not recommend **discography**, but if you are thinking about surgery, you may be asked by the surgeon to undergo this test. Before you do, ask the doctor what information will be gained from the test and what effect it will have on your surgery.

Discography may identify the specific disc level causing pain. It is both a radiographic and therapeutic technique performed by placing a thin needle into a disc, followed by the injection of dye first and anesthetic medication second. The amount of dye required to fill the space, the appearance of the dye in the disc, and reproduction of your back pain are important pieces of information generated by this test. If your back pain is generated by the first injection, a second injection with anesthetic is given in an attempt to relieve your discomfort. Pain relief from medication is also characteristic of a positive test. The test is used to determine the source of back pain when other radiographic techniques have not produced conclusive results.

One of the major problems with discography is its lack of predictive power. The treatment for a positive discography is a bony **fusion** at the level of the disc causing the pain. A study reported on the success of spinal fusion as therapy for a positive discogram versus an unstable spine for spondylolisthesis (see chapter 5). The success rate for the discogenic pain patients was 27 percent. The success rate for the unstable spine patients was 72 percent. Discograms do not predict isolated disc lesions that cause chronic low back pain. There is also a concern that the test itself may hasten the degeneration of discs that undergo discogram procedures.

The procedure is done using a fluoroscope to determine the placement of the needle as it is moved into the disc. The length of the procedure depends on the number of discs studied. Radiation exposure is two rads; the cost is approximately $600.

## BONE DENSITOMETRY

This is a useful way to measure bone mass; low bone mass resulting from a loss of calcium from the bone is associated with increased risk for fracture. **Dual energy X ray absorptiometry** (DXA) is the method most frequently used to determine **bone mineral density** in the spine and the thigh bone. Low-energy X rays are used to determine the difference in the absorption of the beam by the bone versus the soft tissues. Bone tissue will absorb the beam of X rays, whereas X rays will pass through the soft tissues. The difference in absorption corresponds to the amount of calcium in the bones. The best candidates for this test are postmenopausal women, and men and women taking **corticosteroids**.

You will be flat on your back on a table during this test while the arm of the machine passes over you for about twenty to thirty minutes. This test measures both the lumbar spine and hips. The amount of radiation is low, 0.1 rad, and the cost is approximately $280.

Measurement of bone mineral density may also be done by measuring calcium content in the calcaneus, or heel. This is sometimes referred to as a heel DXA. The heel DXA is portable and can be offered to individuals who may not have access to a regular table DXA examination. Debate exists in the medical community whether the heel DXA predicts fracture risk as well as a DXA of the spine and hip. Low bone mineral density on a heel DXA is a sign of osteoporosis. A normal exam is reassuring. However, I recommend that individuals at risk (strong family history of osteoporosis, corticosteroid exposure, for example) go for a full body DXA of the hips and lumbar spine.

## ELECTRODIAGNOSTIC TESTS

Electrodiagnostic tests are useful to confirm the suspicion of nerve compression and are commonly used to evaluate peripheral nerves that travel beyond the spinal cord. These tests are also used to detect muscle and nerve damage; they demonstrate abnormalities in nerve and muscle function but do not identify the specific cause of the dysfunction. Electromyogram (EMG) tests evaluate the electrical activity generated by muscles at rest and at work. Nerve conduction velocity (NCV) studies measure the speed of the transmission of the electrical signal in a nerve. Both of these tests are useful in differentiating among the neurologic disorders associated with back and leg pain. These tests are most often needed to evaluate pain that radiates down the leg (**radiculopathy**).

EMG involves inserting needles into muscles that are supplied by the damaged nerve, as well as other muscles in the back and leg. The process of inserting the needles is painful and requires contracting the muscle after insertion. The amount of irritation and the amount of electricity generated by the muscle help determine the degree of injury to the nerve.

Damage does not occur as soon as the nerve is injured, and abnormalities may take a week or more to appear. For example, disc compression on a nerve may take days before the muscle supplied by that nerve has abnormal electrical signals. Therefore, electrodiagnostic tests done too early will miss the abnormality. EMG tests may take two to four weeks before being helpful. Once a nerve is damaged, the number of nerve fibers supplying a muscle diminishes even if the nerve compression is removed. That change in nerve function, measured by an EMG, may be permanent. No X ray radiation is associated with an EMG test, but it is associated with pain by the insertion of needles into tested muscles. An EMG procedure takes about sixty minutes to complete. The cost ranges from $32 to $376, depending on the number of muscles tested.

NCV studies determine the speed of the signal as it travels through the nerves in the legs or arms. Surface electrodes that look like felt pads are placed over a muscle in the foot. Another pad is placed over the same nerve in a location further up the leg. These pads can be moved over different locations on the limb where the nerve can be pinched by structures in the leg. An electrical signal is generated in the pad closer to the center of the body. The signal is detected at the distal pad and the speed of conduction is matched against normal velocities. Slowing of the speed with which the signal is transferred down the leg determines areas of compression of the nerve outside of the spinal canal. The cost of this test ranges from $58 to $580, depending on the number of nerve conductions tested.

While electrodiagnostic tests document the presence of nerve dysfunction, they do not determine the specific cause. An abnormal EMG documents the location of nerve damage and helps the surgeon identify individuals for whom surgery is likely to bring improvement. NCV differentiates between spinal cord problems and peripheral nerve disorders. I order these tests when I need to determine the exact level of nerve dysfunction in order to provide guidance to anesthesiologists for therapeutic injections or to surgeons for the area of spine surgery.

## BLOOD TESTS

Since most of my patients have mechanical low back pain, which does not cause abnormalities detected in blood tests, these laboratory tests are seldom needed. However, they are necessary when red flags are identified. Only a few blood tests are useful for identifying abnormalities associated with medical back pain. These include an **erythrocyte sedimentation rate** (ESR), **C-reactive protein** (CRP), complete blood count (CBC), and blood chemistries.

ESR is a simple test that measures the speed that red blood cells fall in a tube. Centuries ago, Hippocrates, the Greek physician whom we call the "father of medicine," commented that blood that separated and settled into a clear part and a red part was associated with an ill person. Red blood cells fall because they are coated with an increased level of proteins that are generated because of inflammation anywhere in the body. The inflammation may indicate infection, a tumor, or inflammatory arthritis, which are not mechanical disorders. The normal ESR level is less than 10 mm/hour in men and 20 mm/hour in women. ESR greater than 100 mm/hour is often associated with tumors. ESR may return toward normal as the underlying disorder is treated and improves.

CRP is a protein produced by the liver when inflammation is present, and CRP may rise before the ESR becomes elevated. The normal level of CRP for the standard test is less than 0.2 mg/100 ml. Levels between 1 and 10 mg/100 ml are moderate increases; levels over 10 are markedly elevated. Levels of CRP remain elevated in chronic inflammatory states. Elevated ESR or CRP call for more intense evaluation in order to determine the medical cause of low back pain. High sensitivity CRP (hsCRP) measures lower levels of CRP than measured by the standard test and is ordered to determine risk for cardiovascular disease. Using the same measurement, high risk is associated with 0.3mg/100 ml. These low levels are not significant for the identification of systemic inflammatory diseases.

CBC (red and white blood cells and platelets) and chemistry tests are more often performed to monitor toxicity of drugs than to identify the cause of back pain. Nonsteroidal anti-inflammatory drugs often are prescribed to treat low back pain, and those who take these drugs for an extended period of time are given blood tests to monitor the hematocrit (red blood count) and liver and kidney function.

Medical history, physical examination, and X ray and blood tests allow your doctor to separate mechanical and medical causes of low back pain and set you on the road to recovery—whether with basic care you can provide yourself, or with further medical treatment.

## DR. B'S PRESCRIPTION SUMMARY

- Plain X rays reveal a specific diagnosis in only a small number of back pain sufferers.
- MRI is the best technique to identify soft tissue abnormalities in nerves, bone marrow, and muscles.
- CT scan is the best technique for showing bone abnormalities but is associated with the highest levels of ionizing radiation.
- Bone scan is the best survey technique to evaluate the entire skeleton for abnormal bone activity.
- Anatomic changes identified on radiographic tests become important when they correlate with your back pain complaints.
- Electrodiagnostic tests identify the location of nerve damage.
- Blood tests help distinguish mechanical from medical low back pain.

# Part II

# KNOWING YOUR TREATMENT OPTIONS

# Chapter 4

# The Basic Back Pain Relief Program

MY BASIC THERAPY for low back and leg pain can work for you as long as your pain is not from a systemic illness. Pain from a mechanical disorder such as muscle strain, joint irritation, herniated disc, or hip arthritis, for example, can improve if you control physical activities, use over-the-counter pain medications, stay fit with aerobic exercise, and—most importantly—self-educate. If your back pain improves, you probably won't need any more evaluation to speed your recovery. If you are in doubt about your recovery, contact your physician immediately.

## CONTROL PHYSICAL ACTIVITIES BUT LIMIT BED REST

In the past we were told to lie down if we had back pain, to let the muscles rest and heal. This is wrong! Now we know that bed rest is no better for resolving back pain than being up and walking around. Movement seems to help the tissues of the back heal more rapidly, too. Extended bed rest, on the other hand, deconditions the heart, lungs, stomach, and skeletal muscles. So keep bed rest to a minimum. Studies have shown that two days of bed rest is as good as seven days of bed rest for the relief of back pain. The benefits of bed rest are also limited if pain travels to your leg. In a study of 183 people with sciatica from a herniated disc, people given bed rest for two weeks did no better than those allowed to walk around.

On the other hand, being out of bed does not mean returning to your usual daily work and recreational activities. Stay home from work until you are able to walk or stand for thirty minutes without pain and you feel comfortable sitting for twenty to thirty minutes without increased pain. If you have acute low back pain, limit your activities and you will have a faster recovery and be much less likely to have chronic or recurrent episodes of low back pain. Increase activity as pain decreases.

## Bed Rest Positions

When bed rest is indicated, a couple of positions are most comfortable. The semi-Fowler position places the least pressure on spinal discs, joints, and muscles: put a small pillow behind your head and two to three pillows under your knees to flex your hips and knees. Your mattress should be firm, but it may feel better to lie on a comforter on the floor.

## Get Out of Bed Carefully

Another comfortable position is on your side with a flat back, with your legs curled up with a pillow between your knees. This is a side semi-Fowler position and is the way to get into and out of bed. Push against the bed with your lower arm while letting your legs slide off the edge of the bed. The weight of your legs will swing your chest up with the help of your lower arm. To get back into bed, do the reverse. Shift your upper body weight to the palm of your hand resting on the bed. Slowly let your body down, shifting your weight to your forearm, elbow, and shoulder while you swing your legs up to the bed. Keep your back straight.

## Don't Sleep on Your Stomach

This position is particularly stressing on the lumbar spine because it increases the curve and tends to stretch the muscles in the pelvis, causing more pain. If you have to sleep on your stomach, put a pillow or two under your abdomen. This will flatten your spine and place less pressure on the psoas muscle in the pelvis.

### What Kind of Bed Is Best for Back Pain?

You would think that with as much time as people have been sleeping on beds I would have the answer to this question. What seems to be clear is that preferences are as numerous as the people who go to sleep every night.

When I began my professional career, I thought only a rock-hard bed would be best for back pain patients. Over the years, I have learned that what may be good for a person on one side of the bed may not be so good for the other. How do you solve this dilemma?

There are a wide variety of mattresses constructed with different technologies:

Innerspring—The most common type of mattress. The mattress contains tempered steel coils along with cushioning and insulation. A high coil count or thicker spring does not necessarily make a better bed. What is important is that the springs are individually wrapped (pocketed coil spring technology) that minimizes motion transfer when you move.

Foam—Solid foam mattresses have viscoelastic memory that allows the bed to contour to your body in response to body weight and heat. I find these beds to be best for those people with healthy backs. Many a patient has described "climbing" out of their bed in the morning that causes them more discomfort.

Air technology—These mattresses have air-filled chambers that can inflate or deflate to adjust firmness to your preference. This type of mattress can be modified when your back is well and when it may need to be softer during one of those painful episodes.

Pillowtop—A soft layer of material is sown to the top of the mattress to allow the bed some "give." The soft top over a firm mattress allows for good support while allowing a flattening of the spine.

Water—The days of sloshing back and forth are over. However, this is the form of mattress with the least spine support. I suggest water beds only for those individuals with normal backs.

There are a few ways of testing what makes your back better before buying a bed. The back, between the pelvis and the shoulders, is like an upside down suspension bridge. The supports for this semicircle are the buttocks and shoulders. The firmer the bed, the more the supports will stay above the water and keep tension in the back, maintaining the lumbar curve, or lordosis. The softer the bed, the more the supports will sink, placing less tension on the lumbar spine, causing it to lose the lordosis, or flatten.

The more you want to maintain a lumbar curve, the firmer the mattress you want. If you want to test this idea, try sleeping on a few blankets or an exercise mat on the floor for a few nights. If your back feels rested, a hard mattress is for you. If you prefer a flat back, a softer mattress will do.

I love to swim, but making waves at night was never one of my ideas of how to sleep. Despite my apprehensions about waterbeds, some back pain sufferers swear by them. I do not know how that degree of softness can be helpful to the spine. I believe that, given the choice, those who prefer a flat back will prefer a water bed. Once again, try it out before you buy one.

Some mattresses are reported to contour specifically to your body and support your back no matter what its shape. These mattresses use special foam or air to support the back. Some of my patients have found these to be excellent, while others have found them less desirable. The idea of full support is a good one, but some patients require a firmer surface for comfort.

These suggestions are starting points to decide on your personal preference. You will be sleeping on the bed and need to decide if it will be restful to you. Do not be bashful. Go to the mattress store and test out the merchandise. Rest on them for twenty to thirty minutes to feel if they are comfortable. Having some medical name (chiropractic, orthopedic) associated with the name of the bed does not guarantee that the bed will be good for you. The only way to know is to test it out.

A study examined the bed preferences of individuals who suffered back pain. They had a choice of very firm, moderately firm, and soft mattresses. The winner—moderate firmness. For those individuals with very firm mattresses, using a pillowtop mattress cover is another way of changing the firmness of the mattress at times when your back is bothering you.

## USING OVER-THE-COUNTER MEDICATIONS

The final goal of all therapies is to achieve a back that is painless and functional without drugs. Once maximum function has been reached, medicines can be gradually decreased so you can function without them. But do take them to reduce pain so you can keep moving.

Acetaminophen (Tylenol) is a pure pain reliever (analgesic) without any anti-inflammatory effect. The maximum dose is 4,000 mg per day (six tablets of Tylenol Arthritis). The long-acting form of acetaminophen (650 mg) lasts six to eight hours. Acetaminophen is easily tolerated and doesn't upset your stomach. However, for many people, the medication is not powerful enough to decrease pain.

Nonsteroidal anti-inflammatory drugs (NSAID) have pain-relieving and anti-inflammatory effects. Aspirin was the first NSAID and is still a very powerful drug in adequate doses. For example, patients with rheumatoid arthritis will ingest sixteen tablets a day in divided doses. At this dose it is analgesic and anti-inflammatory. At lower doses, aspirin is analgesic with less anti-inflammatory effects. The problem with aspirin is that it irritates the stomach and can cause ulcers with bleeding. It can also have bad effects on kidney function. At toxic doses, aspirin can cause dizziness, loss of hearing, and even coma. If you take aspirin at a dose higher than 81 mg (baby aspirin) for any length of time, you should be evaluated by a physician.

A number of NSAIDs are available without a prescription:

- Ibuprofen (Advil, Nuprin, Motrin IB)
- Naproxen (Aleve)

The dose for each of these NSAIDs is different, so read the label on the box to determine the effective, safe dose. If one NSAID does not work, try another, because one that helps another person may not help you. If you take an NSAID for two weeks without benefit, then you need to see your doctor. Potential side effects of NSAIDs are that they can cause stomach pain and bleeding, elevations in blood pressure, and decreased function of the kidney in a few people. These drugs need monitoring by your doctor if you take them on a continuous basis.

More potent and more effective NSAIDs are available by prescription. These include a COX-2 inhibitor, which is as effective as the NSAIDs with fewer gastrointestinal side effects.

It is important to understand how long your dose of medicine will be effective, what side effects may occur, and how long you need to remain on a medication. For a full explanation of using drugs for pain, see chapter 9.

## APPLIED THERAPY

### Cold or Heat

Applying cold or heat in the form of ice massage or wet heat, respectively, is a noninvasive way to improve low back pain. Ice massage is used first to decrease swelling and act as an analgesic. Cold decreases the sensitivity of the sensory fibers, blocking the transmission of pain signals. However, cold tends to stiffen muscles and soft tissue. With an acute muscle strain in the lumbar spine, ice massage for the first forty-eight hours is appropriate. Apply an ice pack for about ten minutes and then remove it. Do this a few times a day.

Heat—wet or dry—can improve blood flow and speed healing. Heat can increase muscle flexibility and improve movement. Personal preference tends to drive the decision regarding dry or wet heat. The important point is not to burn your skin. Leave the heat on for ten to fifteen minutes. The maximum safe exposure is thirty minutes. If you have any circulation problems, speak with your doctor about the amount of time your skin should be exposed to temperature extremes.

If my suggestions for cold and heat applications do not seem to be helping, try the opposite temperature. You may feel better with heat early in the course of a back attack. Or you may be one of the people who have greater pain relief with ice massage for chronic low back pain. Some people use both—ice soon after exercise, and heat an hour or two later.

Jane is a spry seventy-two-year-old woman who prefers not to take medicines for her back pain. She prefers to use both ice massage and wet heat for her intermittent back pain. She uses her ice massage for ten minutes at a time when her pain is more intense. The cold has a calming effect on the muscles in her back. She will apply ice three to four times in a day if her pain persists. She will use wet heat when she has stiffness associated with her pain; she applies the heat for about fifteen minutes at a time and will use it three to four times a day. She will use heat and cold when she exercises. To warm up, she will apply some heat to her back. She will apply cold to her back after exercise if it has been particularly strenuous.

### Corsets

Corsets are wide elastic bands with Velcro fasteners. They come in a variety of widths, with or without heat-molded plastic inserts. Some back pain sufferers use corsets for greater stability to the lumbar spine. The rationale is to increase intra-abdominal pressure in order to decrease the stress on the lumbar spine. Corsets do not keep your lumbar spine motionless. They do remind you to use your legs when lifting, which may be the most important effect of wearing a corset. The downside is that use of a corset will make your muscles weak, so persistent use can be counterproductive. You could be at greater risk of having a back attack.

Wear a corset when you are at risk for excessive strain on your spine, such as with heavy lifting or sitting for long periods of time. Many workers are given corsets to help them when doing heavy physical labor. In my experience when I was working in the hospital, the physical plant staff had their corsets flapping in the breeze. They did not close them because they were too constricting. Also, corsets may constrict blood vessels in the abdomen and can increase blood pressure. Take off the corset as soon as you are out of your risky situation. You must be committed to strengthening exercises once you take off your corset to maintain your back muscles. You should also be aware that wearing a corset can raise blood pressure

Some patients with kyphosis (chest forward bend) will wear a brace with straps that go over the shoulders. The amount of backward force on the spine depends on the amount of tension on the straps. Lucy is a sixty-eight-year-old woman with a forward posture that will cause her pain toward the end of the day. She has a brace with shoulder straps that she wears when she is going to be standing for any length of time. The gentle pressure on her spine allows her to stand for a length of time that would not be imaginable without support.

## AEROBICS: EXPANDING YOUR COMFORT ZONE—GRADUALLY

Aerobic exercises that improve endurance can help back pain as discomfort starts to decrease. How will you know that you are improving? You will notice that you will feel more comfortable for increasing amounts of time out of bed. You will be able to walk longer distances around your house and outside. As you get better, you will be able to sit for longer periods of time without feeling tired.

Choose an exercise program that you will continue over an extended period of time and something that is easily accessible. You may love to swim, but if there's no pool nearby, this program is not realistic. Exercises most helpful for low back pain are walking, swimming, or riding a stationary bicycle. Before your back pain began, you may have been running instead of walking, or swimming timed laps instead of paddling in the pool, or riding a regular bicycle. I am frequently asked, "How much exercise can I do?" The question is best answered with an explanation of the "Comfort Zone."

## Comfort Zone

Exercise makes muscles more efficient and the key to successful training is to use muscles without damaging muscle cells. With damage, the muscles must heal for longer periods of time. This is counterproductive. Finding the fine line between stressing your muscles and causing damage can be difficult. I try to guide my patients to find a happy medium with the concept of the Comfort Zone.

If you have been exercising and have developed low back pain, cut back your exercise to one-tenth of what you were doing before the pain started. For example, if you were walking ten blocks, you would cut back your exercise to one block. You might say that is no exercise at all, but that amount of exercise would be in the Comfort Zone. You would do the exercise and would feel no additional soreness the next day. That means you are able to do the exercise safely without causing any damage to the stressed muscles.

Then, every other day increase your exercise another block or another minute. As you increase your effort you will gradually move toward the Margin Zone. In this zone, the muscles stay sore for a longer period of time measured in hours, but less than a single day. At this point, cut back your exercise slightly to the previous level that did not cause increased soreness. Continue training at the lower level of effort until no soreness remains at the end of the exercise. At that point, the Comfort Zone of exercise has been expanded. Increases in times or repetitions are slowed at this point so that your training is between the Comfort Zone and the Margin Zone. Over time you will expand your Comfort Zone to increasing levels of exercise.

The goal of this slow progression is to get the benefits of exercise without falling into the Discomfort Zone. This is where discomfort may last for extended periods of time measured in days. Exercises are discontinued entirely until muscle pain from the exercise has resolved. The trouble with being in this zone is determining the amount of exercise that is safe. It may have been at one block or ten blocks. You cannot tell. That is why starting out in the Comfort Zone is so important.

This basic concept can work for any form of exercise—the treadmill, the stair climber, or strength machines. Start out with an amount of exercise that is safe. Once you know that you can complete the exercise without increasing your pain, you can quickly increase your exercise without causing a relapse. I have seen many patients improve with this guidance for their exercise. Try these concepts. I know that you will gain the benefits of exercise with much less risk for reinjury.

### The Elusive Last 10 Percent of Recovery

After a while, you will have achieved a significant improvement in your condition with a combination of therapies. Your level of improvement may allow your return to work and most of your recreational activities. However, let's say you have a specific activity that you enjoy. This may be hiking five miles, playing three sets of tennis, or running twenty miles per week. Your activity improvement may be 85 or 90 percent of your original state before back pain occurred. This level of improvement may mean that you are able to hike, but only four miles. Your tennis games may be shorter and less frequent. Your running may be sixteen miles on the track at the high school. Your function is not as good as it was prior to your episode of back pain—but it is in the Comfort Zone. Some people who have had this improvement are not satisfied with their function. They search for the final 10 percent of function. They want to be exactly as they were prior to their back episode.

The problem is that this final 10 percent can be difficult to achieve. The search for this complete recovery is as successful as the quest for the Holy Grail. I have seen many patients search for that one elusive therapy that will restore them to their original state. They concentrate on what is lost versus what they have regained. They end up disappointed. Their pessimistic attitude makes it more difficult to reach their goal. People who accept their improvement and work from that point have a better chance of having a positive outcome. Think about it.

## MAINTAIN A POSITIVE ATTITUDE

You may not believe it, but just learning about the causes of back pain and the fact that it gets better on its own has a great therapeutic effect. The positive feelings that come from knowing that your problem will be solved heal low back pain. Understanding the cause of your back pain goes a long way in relieving your anxiety concerning the potential threat to your health. The relief of stress plays an important role in the resolution of back pain, whether acute or chronic. Such knowledge is as powerful as **manipulation** by a chiropractor or exercises supervised by a physical therapist.

In a study conducted in the state of Washington, researchers assigned 321 people who had back pain for seven days or less to an exercise program supervised by physical therapists, to manipulation treatments given by chiropractors, or to an educational booklet about low back pain. In the first month of the study, the people in the exercise and manipulation programs had less pain. However, at one year, no differences could be found concerning days lost from work or the frequency of additional attacks of low back pain among the groups. The cost of the educational booklet was one-third of the expense of the exercise and manipulation therapies. Knowledge is an affordable way to treat low back pain. The people informed about their back pain with the educational booklet needed to go to the doctor less frequently than those who received no information.

You can learn about back pain from this book and others, from videotapes and audiotapes on back exercises, and from the Internet. But be careful on the Internet. There's a great deal of wrong information there, so know the reputation of the group presenting the information. I have listed a number of Internet sites from well-regarded professional groups in appendix C. These websites are updated on a regular basis to offer current information.

One of my patients has taught me the power of a positive attitude. She is ill with a multitude of medical problems, any one of which could devastate a negative person. She returns to my office on a regular basis. She is always nicely dressed and has a smile on her face despite chronic pain and disability. I asked her what her secret was. How in the face of all these difficulties, the chronic nature of her illness, the multiple medicines she needs to take to function, does she continue with such a positive attitude? She told me her secret was very simple. Long ago when her problems started to mount up, she made a choice. She said, "I can be better or bitter. I decided to concentrate on the e and not the i." She is a testimonial to the therapeutic powers of a positive attitude. Be positive and you can be better even in the face of adversity.

## IF BACK PAIN IS CHRONIC

The therapy for chronic low back pain is more complicated. The goal of therapy is maximizing function despite some continued pain. Pain may be exacerbated at times, but this is not necessarily indicative of past or present disease-associated damage.

Chronic back pain can be treated with basic therapy for acute low back pain. But basic therapy is only occasionally fully effective. Other therapies are added to this basic program. Many of the medications used for the treatment of chronic pain are not specifically pain relievers. These agents tend to have effects on other functions of the nervous system. Many times a medicine that is indicated for a nonpain problem is used in people who have chronic pain. Their pain is relieved. That is one of the ways multiple uses for medicines are discovered. For example, gabapentin (Neurontin) is a medicine used for the control of a kind of seizure. Some of these same patients had chronic pain that was eased while taking gabapentin. Subsequently, gabapentin was given to patients who did not have seizures but who had pain relief with the medicine. Another group of medicines that help chronic pain are the antidepressants. Tricyclic antidepressants (amitriptyline, for example) are sometimes used to increase the chemicals that stimulate the pain inhibitory pathway. Other classes of antidepressants, like duloxitene (Cymbalta), also help relieve chronic pain. As an added feature, these drugs help with the depression that accompanies chronic pain.

If you continue to experience pain, try counterirritant therapy such as TENS, massage, or acupuncture. The relaxation response may decrease the stress associated with chronic pain. Therapies that can result in a relaxation response include **yoga**, **biofeedback**, and hypnosis. You and your physician need to meet on a regular basis to modify your therapies to obtain the best outcome.

### Control Better Than Cure

Some of you reading this book might believe curing a problem is better than controlling it. In all honesty, a cure in human biology is very difficult to achieve. Except for bacterial infections, most human diseases are controlled, not cured. This applies to back pain, too. You may have no pain and function normally. You may think you are cured. However, you are at much greater risk for a second episode of back pain within the next year. That suggests that your back problem has not been cured.

The constant monitoring that comes with controlling a medical problem is a better way to deal with low back pain. Control suggests that you will need to continue to exercise in an appropriate manner to maintain the strength of your back. Although it takes more work on your part, controlling your condition will make you ready to remedy any hint of back pain as soon as it appears.

Despite the best efforts of the human body to heal, many of you will not be better at two, three, or four weeks after the start of an attack of low back pain. Your pain has persisted in the area of the low back, with radiation no farther than the buttock or back of the upper leg. In those circumstances, a visit to a physician is important for an evaluation and additional therapy. As opposed to other health care professionals, a physician is the appropriate practitioner to go to for evaluation and therapy first. Physicians have access to all the diagnostic tools to determine what is wrong with your back. They also have the ability to prescribe all the conventional and complementary therapies that can help acute low back pain. You can read about all of these therapies in the following chapters.

---

### DR. B'S PRESCRIPTION SUMMARY

- Rest in bed only if you have leg pain. Otherwise, limit bed rest and walk as much as you can tolerate.
- Try over-the-counter **analgesics** and nonsteroidal anti-inflammatory drugs (NSAIDs).
- As your back pain begins to resolve, do low-impact aerobic exercise such as walking or swimming.
- Do not exercise your back too soon after the beginning of a back pain episode. Certain back exercises can increase pain if you do them too early in the healing process. Expand your Comfort Zone gradually.
- Maintain a positive attitude and educate yourself about your back. This positive attitude has a beneficial effect on your healing. Remember most back pain resolves in two months. Don't assume you will be the exception.
- Knowledge is power. Knowing that you will get better, makes you better.

# Chapter 5

# Recognizing and Treating
# Mechanical Low Back Pain

MOST BACK PAIN is due to mechanical causes, such as muscle strain and trauma, disc degeneration and arthritis, herniated discs and sciatica, spinal stenosis and scoliosis. While my basic back pain relief program helps most back pain, it is important to know when you have a condition that may require more extensive medical treatment.

## MUSCLE STRAIN, SPASM, AND TRAUMA

Back strain is injury to muscles, fascia, ligaments, or tendons and is one of the most common causes of low back pain. Everyday events cause back strain. You can cough or sneeze and cause this strain, or you can lift an object heavier than your muscles and ligaments can support. Or you can engage in a perfectly ordinary motion like bending over to pick up a sock.

Regardless of cause, the damage to the back tissues results in a reflex signal sent through the local nervous system, thereby alerting all the muscles supplied by the nerve that one of the stations in the network has been damaged. This alert protects the injured muscle and results in a muscle spasm, which tightens all the muscles in the network even though only one muscle was injured.

This muscle spasm in the lumbar spinal muscles is much like a charley horse that may develop when you run, ski, or swim. While severity varies, the pain can be overwhelming—you may have seen an Olympic runner actually fall to the ground as a result of a charley horse. Sometimes the muscle spasm is immobilizing and the person can't move at all. These muscle traumas are relatively common when bodies aren't well prepared for strenuous activity.

Ben, forty-two, came to see me with a typical winter story. A February snowstorm had dropped about eight inches of snow on his driveway, and he had to shovel it off before it hardened into ice. Because he played tennis in the summer months and walked on his treadmill during the winter, he thought he was in good shape. However, he did no weight lifting, and he went out to shovel the snow without warming up his muscles or wearing adequate outdoor clothing. Ten minutes into his shoveling job, he picked up a particularly heavy load of snow and twisted his body to the left to place it in a new pile. Before he could straighten his body, he felt severe pain in the right side of his low back, and the muscles in his back tightened as he stood there. With great effort, he managed to get into his house and get into bed, where, incidentally, his pain increased. The next day, Ben called to say that his back was so stiff he could not move. I told him to get out of bed and slowly and carefully walk around his house. Over time, Ben improved with a combination of exercises and nonprescription medications. However, this bout with pain made him promise himself that from then on, he would hire neighborhood kids to shovel his driveway.

### Relaxing Muscles

Muscle tightness may accompany any disorder that causes pain in the lumbar spine. Muscle spasms occur in order to reduce motion and decrease irritation to the injured structures, and the best way to relieve spasms is to keep moving. Incremental—gradual—motions relieve spasm and allow the muscle to continuously test how far it can stretch. As the irritation is relieved, the muscles will go back to their normal tension. Remember this point, however: the first place to be injured will be the last to improve.

In addition to gradual motion, medications (aspirin-like medicines), cold packs (to relieve pain initially), a heating pad (to improve blood flow later), and stretching exercises are all appropriate self-care treatments to relieve the discomfort of back strain. Not all of these therapies are necessarily required, however, and you may respond to any one component (see chapter 4).

Muscle relaxants can offer relief for muscle spasms that are severe. I have found these drugs to be particularly effective for individuals who have muscle spasms that do not respond to pain relievers and stretching exercises. The big concern about muscle relaxants is the side effect of sleepiness. Muscle relaxants can be effective without causing sleepiness. In fact only a small number of people have sleepiness when taking muscle relaxants. However, you should not drive a car or engage in an activity that requires your full attention when you first start taking these medicines. You need to be sure that you are not one of the minority of people who get sleepy from these drugs. You should ask your doctor about the addition of a muscle relaxant if you have experienced tight muscles in the low back. Muscle relaxants may be effective for you even if you have had muscle spasms for weeks or months without improvement.

## DISC DEGENERATION AND OSTEOARTHRITIS (LUMBAR SPONDYLOSIS)

After age thirty, your discs become less effective cushions; they start to resemble pancakes. In addition, loss of spacing puts more pressure on the facet joints at the back of the vertebrae, a process that results in lumbar **spondylosis**. These degenerative changes occur in all of us as we age, but in some of us they happen sooner.

Facet joints normally allow motion forward and backward and do not carry weight, but as the cushioning of the discs lessens, more and more body weight is placed on the facet joints. When the facet joints begin bearing weight, they start wearing out. These changes eventually lead to **osteoarthritis**, the most common form of arthritis; osteoarthritis often also involves the knee or hip.

Narrowing discs and changes in the facet joints may be a painless process, but it may also cause severe localized back pain. Individual differences are the rule, and we can't predict who will have pain associated with lumbar spondylosis. X rays and MRIs can detect changes in the joints and the degenerative discs, but these tests are unable to predict future pain. This is important because many patients come to me with MRIs demonstrating disc degeneration, but these changes may be inconsequential. Discogram procedures are reported as positive but are not reliable at identifying offending disc levels. As mentioned, a number of studies have shown that people with no complaints or history of back pain may show significant disc degeneration when given radiographic tests. On the other hand, osteoarthritis of the facet joints can cause significant back pain that requires attention in order to improve.

## Facet Syndrome

Facet joints may cause increasing pain as they degenerate. These joints can cause pain that is present in the low back only. This pain is made worse with standing or bending backward or to the side and is relieved with sitting. However, as the degeneration progresses, the nerves to the joints become increasingly irritated and send signals along the "computer network" attached to that facet joint. This is referred pain that was described in chapter 1. The signals in the network can cause muscles in the low back, thigh, or calf to be tight. Pain may be experienced in the buttock, hamstring area, and lower leg. The longer the pain remains a problem, the less likely that sitting or bending forward will relieve the pain.

Almost everybody with lumbar spondylosis improves with nonsurgical therapy.

Appliances—artificial discs—designed to replace discs in the spine remain in a developmental and experimental stage. We need many more years of testing before disc replacements will be available to the small group of patients with intractable back pain related to degenerative disc disease. In fact, the presence of osteoarthritis in the facet joints eliminates you as an appropriate recipient of an artificial disc replacement.

## Treatment for Spondylosis with Exercise and Medications

Disc degeneration and osteoarthritis are primarily treated with exercises. If you limit the motion of your spine, stiffness and fatigue often result. Stiffness and fatigue are sources of pain in the low back. Range-of-motion exercises help maintain movement of the spine. Add medication if physical function is limited by increasing local back pain. Osteoarthritis of the lumbar spine is treated with analgesics, NSAIDs, and muscle relaxants in varying combinations.

Many patients are concerned about getting started with medicines. They believe that they will become "addicted" to the drugs and will never get off of them. I tell my patients that taking medicine is not the goal of therapy. The drugs are used to "facilitate function." You may hurt too much to even begin an exercise program. Medicines allow that initial effort to start an exercise program. The nonopioid medicines have no addictive properties. You will use medicine until you have improved your function. You will then use medicine as you need. You are in control. You know what works and how to use it.

## Traction Therapy: Stretching You Out

Traction therapy was a common therapy given to hospitalized individuals in the 1950s. Patients were fitted with a brace with straps that were attached to weights that were hung off the end of the bed. More times than not, the patients extricated themselves from the contraptions to go the bathroom. Traction therapy was at least a way of getting patients in the hospital resting. Of course, we have come to understand that prolonged bed rest is not good therapy for back pain. Traction was never proven to be helpful.

More recently, traction therapy has had a comeback with dynamic systems that pull on the back in cycles instead of a constant pressure. The principle behind these systems is that the negative pressure on the discs and joints increase the flow if nutrients into these structures allowing for healing.

However, in studies looking at therapeutic versus sham traction, the benefits were the same in both groups. What may have been of greatest benefit was the graded exercise program used by both groups. Getting on the rack is not as helpful as you doing exercises.

## Facet Joint Injection for Osteoarthritis

If you have osteoarthritis, you will likely respond to oral drugs and will not need additional therapies. But you may be one of the few who have increased pain when bending to the side. The location of this side-bending pain does not change and is just off to the side of the middle of the back. These symptoms are characteristic of arthritis that affects the facet joints. When other therapies are ineffective, facet joint injections help decrease the pain.

The chance for success is increased when the injections are done with the help of X rays so that the needle can be placed exactly in the joint. Under fluoroscopic guidance, the injection of anesthetic and corticosteroid decreases the inflammation of the joint. In addition, the nerves supplying sensation to this joint (medial branch) can be numbed by injection. The beneficial effect of the injection can last from days to months. The injections can be repeated every two months.

A more permanent, but more invasive, method to decrease pain in the facet joint is by facet **neurotomy**. This procedure uses heat (**radiofrequency**) or cold (**cryoablation**) to damage nerves supplying sensation to the facet joints. The point of the therapy is destruction of the nerves to the facet joint by searing or freezing them. We expect that the procedure will destroy all the nerves that cause the pain, without damaging any of the nerves supplying the muscles.

These procedures require you to be awake while the injections are given. Even when the procedure is done properly, all the sources of pain may not be reached. In addition, the procedure itself has the potential to cause increased low back pain. Therefore, I add these procedures as part of a complete prescription in only the most severe cases of **facet syndrome** that have been resistant to NSAIDs, muscle relaxants, exercises, and long-acting opioids.

Paula is a fifty-eight-year-old woman with facet syndrome. She had oral medicines and an exercise program that was not successful at controlling her facet joint pain that radiated down her leg with standing. She underwent facet joint blocks with numbing medicines that relieved pain on two occasions that identified the joints causing her problem. She had a radiofrequency ablation that has relieved her pain for over two years. She would be a candidate for a repeat procedure if her pain returns.

### Osteoarthritis of the Hip

Arthritis of any type that affects the hip can cause groin pain. Nerves that supply sensation to the hip also innervate the muscles in the low back and thigh. Pain from the hip may also radiate down to the knee, and hip disease may show up as low back or thigh pain. If you have hip arthritis, you may have difficulty walking and you may attribute this to your back.

At fifty-five, Ellen, an attorney, had had difficulty walking for about six months. Her pain was localized to the right buttock and low back, and although she couldn't remember when her pain had started, she'd noticed a gradual increase in the severity of her symptoms. She had been to two other physicians who had focused attention on her lumbar spine as the cause of her symptoms, although X rays and an MRI scan of her spine did not reveal abnormalities. Despite lack of lumbar spine difficulties, her back pain increased and she had more and more trouble getting out of a chair or out of bed in the morning. Ellen's pain also had a detrimental effect on her sexual relationship with her husband because she had trouble finding a comfortable position during sex, one that did not cause more right buttock pain.

She had normal range of motion in her back, but when her right hip was moved by rotating her foot away from the center of her body, she experienced her "back" pain. An X ray taken of the pelvis, as opposed to the lumbar spine, revealed significant joint space narrowing and extra bone formation. When asked if she'd had trauma to this hip in the past, this limping lawyer remembered a horseback riding accident in which she had fallen on that hip but had only a bad bruise and no fracture. This old injury was the probable source of her current problems. I suggested treatment with exercises to strengthen her leg and anti-inflammatory medications. Currently, Ellen is walking without a limp, but she may be a candidate for hip replacement in the future.

## HERNIATED DISC AND SCIATICA

In medical terms, a herniated disc is a rupture of the **nucleus pulposus**—the gel center—through the annulus fibrosus, the outer tire of the intervertebral discs (fig. 5.1). In popular language this is frequently referred to by the misnomer "slipped disc." But discs do not slip. They herniate.

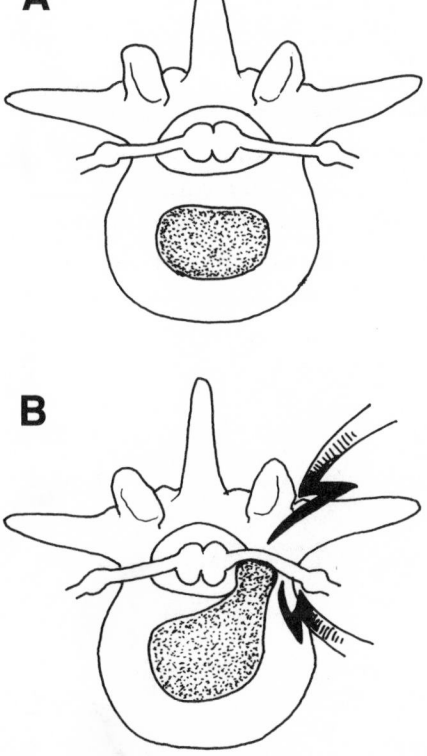

Figure 5.1. In a normal disc (A), the gel center stays in the center of the disc. In a herniated disc (B), the gel center has escaped from its covering and has invaded the spinal canal to compress the spinal nerve.

Most disc ruptures occur between the ages of thirty or forty, a time when discs contain a normal amount of gel and the outer tire is starting to wear out. The gel may remain inside the tire, which is a disc protrusion, or may escape outside the tire entirely, which is a disc extrusion. Extruded pieces of disc may move up or down the spinal canal, and discs may protrude to the front, the sides, or to the back (see fig. 5.1).

Protruded or extruded discs may not be painful unless they irritate the spinal nerves in the spinal canal. The body recognizes the abnormal position of the disc and tries to remove the abnormality. Inflammation that develops when the extruded piece of disc is recognized as "foreign tissue" in the spinal canal may be greater than inflammation that develops when there is a simple protrusion. The release of activated enzymes slowly dissolves the herniated portion of the disc but may also inflame the nearby nerve. Once the nerve is inflamed, sciatica (radicular pain) is generated in the leg.

Sciatica caused by a herniated nucleus pulposus usually leads to leg pain that becomes worse with sitting and improved with standing or lying flat in bed with a pillow under the knees. In many instances, sciatica is preceded by a history of intermittent episodes of low back pain at which time the outer tire of the disc is stretched and under tension. Low back pain may decrease once the disc herniates because the outer tire is no longer under tension. Then low back pain is replaced with pain running to the leg and foot. This pain corresponds to the inflamed nerve caused by the gel from the disc pressing on the nerve.

Morning is the time of day most associated with increased forces on the disc because your discs absorb water during the night while you are lying flat. As mentioned in chapter 1, you are taller in the morning and shorter at the end of the day as gravity pushes water out of your discs, thereby making them thinner.

Any disc in the lumbar spine may rupture, but the ones at the bottom of the lumbar spine herniate most frequently because they carry a greater proportion of the weight of the body. Lumbar disc levels L3, L4, and L5 each correspond to a nerve that affects a different part of your leg or foot. Knowing the part of the leg or foot that is numb or weak helps identify the location of the inflamed nerve.

- The L3–L4 level nerve runs to the thigh and affects the knee. L4 creates loss of sensation in front of your thigh. Weakness occurs in the front and back of your knee. There is a loss of knee reflex.

- The L4–L5 level nerve runs to your big toe and involves sensation loss in front of your lower leg. The big toe becomes weak, causing a foot drop when walking on your heel, No loss of reflex is associated with this disc level.
- The L5–S1 level nerve effects the calf muscle and the bottom of the foot with weakness and loss of sensation from your calf to the outer three toes. There is reflex loss in your ankle.

These patterns are strongly correlated with the level of disc herniation and nerve compression. It is so characteristic that additional evaluation with X rays or an MRI is not necessary to initiate treatment for sciatica.

A progression of abnormalities in the nervous system corresponds to the inflamed nerve—from having no abnormalities to a loss of reflex and sensation to, finally, muscle weakness. You lose sensation before your leg becomes weak because the part of the nerve that attaches to muscles is deep inside the nerve and is surrounded on the outside by the sensory portion of the nerve. If you stretch your leg, the inflamed nerve causes pain down your leg. If you move your leg while lying flat, there will be a point where the affected nerve increases pain. In this flat position, bending your foot toward your head worsens the sciatica.

Pain is deep and sharp and progresses from the back downward in the involved leg, but sciatica may vary in intensity. You may experience pins and needles, or a burning sensation, typical to radicular pain. The pain may be so severe that your back is "locked," or you experience just a dull ache that increases with movement. Pain worsens when you bend forward and improves with bending backward. Characteristically, people with herniated discs have pain with sitting, driving, walking, coughing, sneezing, and having a bowel movement. They have great difficulty bending forward because tightness in the muscles limits motion. Walking is difficult because the affected leg will not move forward in a normal manner, and the leg seems unable to hold your weight.

A herniated disc at a higher level in the lumbar spine can also cause anterior thigh pain, and an evaluation with a physician who will listen to your problem is important. No one physician can take care of all the problems that are associated with anterior thigh pain. However, your physician should be able to identify the general category of the problem and refer you to another physician with the expertise to evaluate and treat your disorder.

## Herniated Disc: Treatment without Surgery

Many studies report a good outcome with nonsurgical medical therapy in 80 percent or more of people with a herniated disc who are followed for five years. The primary element of treatment is movement, although for the first several days after the onset of sciatica, bed rest may be necessary to decrease pain.

Lying flat on your back with a pillow under your legs or resting on your side with a pillow placed between your legs takes tension off the inflamed nerve and decreases pressure on the herniated disc. As soon as possible, however, you should start walking on a flat surface. Stairs must be done with extreme care because of leg weakness.

Drug therapy in the form of anti-inflammatory drugs, muscle relaxants, and opioids are helpful. The NSAIDs are a mainstay of therapy for acute herniated discs with nerve compression because of their anti-inflammatory and analgesic properties. The inflammation involving the nerve is a major cause of leg pain; NSAIDs decrease inflammation surrounding the disc and nerve, thereby reducing pain.

Hal, forty-five, a Washington lobbyist, told me his pain started when he lifted some heavy luggage after a business trip. Within two days he developed back pain that started to radiate into his left thigh. He then noticed an area of numbness over the top of his thigh and a slight imbalance when he went up or down the stairs. His examination revealed normal muscle strength, loss of pinprick sensation over the front of the thigh, the loss of the L4 reflex at the knee, and pain that ran down the front of the thigh with raising the leg, a positive straight leg raising test.

Hal's exam was consistent with a disc herniation at the L3–L4 level, with impingement of the L4 nerve root on the left. Hal had the option of an MRI scan, but I suggested that the scan would not alter the recommended therapy at the initial stage of this disorder, unless he developed greater weakness. He was pleased to hear that an MRI scan was not necessary, since he seemed to pale at the idea of getting into the close quarters of the scanner.

Hal was treated with a combination of Voltaren XR (an NSAID) twice a day, prednisone (a corticosteroid), and oxycodone (an opioid pain reliever) up to four pills per day for pain, and an extension exercise program. Within ten days, his back and thigh pain started to improve. His reflex took about eight weeks to return, and his numbness took about three months to resolve. Gradually Hal stopped his medications; first his opioid pain relievers, then the prednisone, and finally the Voltaren. At five months he had minimal pain in his back if he stood for an extended period.

### Herniated Disc: Indications for Surgery

In certain cases, surgery to remove the portion of the disc that is pressing on the nerve may be indicated. However, indications for surgery are not always clear-cut, which makes the decision difficult for many people. For the rare person with loss of bladder or bowel function (**cauda equina** compression syndrome, or CEC) associated with a large disc herniation, surgery is the only choice.

The other indication for early surgery is progressive muscle weakness. If your foot is in a dropped position and cannot be raised (foot drop), or the thigh muscle will not contract, surgical intervention must be considered. While you may recover from this situation, the process may take an extended period of time. Factors that play a role in the decision process include your pain tolerance, emotional response, work demands, and other lifestyle issues. Studies have shown that individuals who do not improve with medical therapy within the first six weeks improve more quickly with surgery than with an additional course of drug therapy.

Remember the following statement that applies to the vast majority of people with back pain: lumbar spine disc surgery is done for leg pain, not back pain. This statement is important because lumbar spine surgery relieves compression on nerves causing sciatica, leg pain. The surgery is done in the lumbar spine, and no matter what technique is used, the lumbar spine is injured during surgery.

Once the compression is removed, sciatica will resolve. If the appropriate disc level has been decompressed, the pain resolves quickly, with numbness improving over a longer period of time. What surgery often does is make an intolerable condition tolerable (see chapter 12).

Studies have demonstrated that when comparing disc surgery with medical therapy, operations improve your symptoms more rapidly. However, at two years both groups have about the same level of improvement. Studies done over a longer period in patients who have been observed for twenty-five years show that patients who have surgery are at a slightly increased risk of having additional disc herniations compared to disc patients who have used medical therapy. A small proportion have additional spine surgeries compared to the medically treated groups. All these factors need to be considered when making a decision about spine surgery.

## PIRIFORMIS SYNDROME

The piriformis muscle is located deep inside the buttock. The muscle has its origin on the sacral vertebrae and stretches to insert on the thighbone. The muscle works to rotate the thigh laterally. The sciatic nerve runs under the piriformis muscle as it leaves the spinal canal and goes through the sciatic notch and travels down the leg.

Any disorder that irritates the piriformis muscle will cause it to contract, thereby compressing the sciatic nerve. This compression causes a diffuse pain down the leg that follows no single nerve. This characteristic differentiates piriformis syndrome from nerve compression associated with a herniated disc. With piriformis syndrome, you may have difficulty walking because of leg pain. Women may experience vaginal and pelvic pain during sexual intercourse. The pain is made worse when the muscle is stretched, as in bringing the bent leg across the center of the body.

Electrodiagnostic tests will document nerve compression in the area of the buttock, and an MRI scan may detect an enlarged muscle inside the pelvis.

Therapy includes stretching exercises, analgesics, anti-inflammatory medications, and muscle relaxants. With persistent pain, injections of local anesthetics and corticosteroids in the muscles may help (see chapter 9).

John is a fifty-eight-year-old gentleman who happened to sit awkwardly on one buttock for an extended period of time at a sporting event. Later that evening he experienced increasing pain in the buttock with a searing pain down the leg. He had no back pain. The pain was so severe that he was unable to sit. He could stand but lying down caused increased pain making it difficult to sleep. He was evaluated and was found to have increasing pain in the leg when moving the knee toward the center of his body. He had classic signs of piriformis syndrome. He was treated with an NSAID, muscle relaxant, mild pain reliever, and an intense physical therapy program. Gradually, he was able to sleep through the night, and was able to sit for longer time periods. Six weeks was the time required to remedy his piriformis syndrome.

## CRACKED VERTEBRAL BODIES
## (SPONDYLOLYSIS AND SPONDYLOLISTHESIS)

Cartilage plates allow for the growth of bone while we are young, and one such plate exists in the lamina of the vertebrae between the joints. As we mature, our bones become solid and these cartilage plates close. **Spondylolysis** and spondylolisthesis occur because of a crack in this back section of a vertebra.

If physical activities during childhood, such as gymnastics, which involves bending backward, cause enough strain on this cartilage plate, the plate will not close. This is a spondylolysis. If enough strain is placed on the cartilage plate, then the front end of the vertebra, which is no longer attached to the back part of the vertebra, may move forward, and that instability is a spondylolisthesis, commonly known as a slipped vertebra (see fig. 5.2). This instability occurs most frequently at the L5 interspace. Because these spinal abnormalities occur during active growth during childhood, they are called developmental spondylolisthesis. For some, this instability remains painless throughout life. Even physically active individuals, such as football players, may remain free of pain. You may be unaware of the presence of a spondylolisthesis, but it may be identified by chance when an X ray is taken of the abdomen or spine for another reason.

Another form of spondylolisthesis occurs as we age and develops because the facet joints change their shape. This means that the facet joints can't keep the spine in its normal position, and therefore these joints allow slippage forward or backward. This problem, called degenerative spondylolisthesis, is a form of spinal osteoarthritis and occurs most commonly at L4.

Figure 5.2. Spondylolisthesis—a break in the vertebra allows forward slippage.

Lumbar spondylolisthesis is characterized by an unstable spine. The front of the spine, the vertebral body, does not attach to the back of the spine, the facet joints. In most people the ligaments and muscles support the spine without abnormal motion. However, some people have abnormal movement of the spine with standing and they feel better in a forward posture. Back pain, with or without leg pain, occurs as the slippage becomes more significant, at which point you need to limit heavy lifting; therapy includes bracing and strengthening exercises.

Spondylolisthesis presents fewer symptoms while you sit and more pain when you stand, and generally the hamstring muscles are tight. In severe spondylolisthesis, an indentation in the lower lumbar spine is visible.

Usually, adult spondylolysis does not require therapy. However, when necessary, symptomatic spondylolisthesis can be treated with flexion exercises (bending forward), bracing to support the spine, and anti-inflammatory medications to decrease pain. When bracing is unable to control pain, lumbar spine surgery (bony fusion) is necessary, but this is rare. This operation can be very useful to the younger spondylolisthesis patients with persistent low back pain and failure of drug and bracing therapy (see chapters 8 and 10).

## SPINAL STENOSIS

As the space in the spinal canal decreases, more compression is placed on the nerves within the canal. This results in narrowing (stenosis). Disc degeneration and osteoarthritis of the lumbar spine cause a decrease in the room inside the spinal canal. Some fortunate people are born with larger spinal canals, but others have canals with a shape that from an early age diminishes the space in the spine.

Structures that take up room in the spinal canal include extra bone around the joints (osteophytes), degenerative discs, and folded ligaments that line the interior of the spinal canal (ligamentum flavum). Lumbar stenosis may occur in the center or side of the spinal canal or the foramen opening for the nerve root. These areas of spinal canal compression are correlated with pain in different locations in the legs:

- Central stenosis causes pain in one or both legs with walking.
- Lateral stenosis causes pain down one leg with standing.

- Stenosis of a neural foramen causes leg pain that is persistent, regardless of the position.

### Vascular Claudication

Decreased arterial blood flow to the leg (vascular **claudication**) must be differentiated from leg pain that is secondary to spinal stenosis (neurogenic claudication). Vascular claudication, which is one of the important symptoms of cardiovascular disease, causes leg pain with activities such as walking or running. Standing without walking does not cause pain with vascular claudication. A bicycle test is one of the ways to differentiate vascular from neural claudication. If you have neurogenic claudication from spinal stenosis, you can ride a bicycle without leg pain. If you have vascular claudication, exercising on a stationary bicycle will result in leg pain causing you to stop.

Pain associated with spinal stenosis may case back, buttock, thigh, lower leg, or foot pain. The pain may come in any combination of locations from the low back to the foot. You may feel pain only in your leg and none in your back. In addition to pain, you may also have numbness, unusual sensations like tingling (paresthesias), and weakness in the lower extremities. People with spinal stenosis are able to ride a stationary bicycle or walk up stairs or an incline without difficulty. However, standing or walking down the stairs or down an incline causes pain. Spinal stenosis causes leg pain while walking or standing because this posture causes a narrowing of the volume of the spinal canal and stops the blood flow to the spinal nerves. This posture may cause direct pressure on the nerves by structures in the canal including joints, ligaments, or discs. When you bend forward or sit down, your posture increases the volume in the canal, and restores blood flow to the nerve.

Because stenosis can occur at multiple levels of the spine, and more than one level may be causing your leg pain, careful correlation between your symptoms and radiographic findings is essential to determine the critical areas of stenosis. This is the time where electrodiagnostic testing may be helpful in separating central from peripheral nerve disorders, as well as determining the level of central nerve involvement.

Sometimes symptoms of lumbar spinal stenosis are unusual. Early in my medical career, Evan, sixty-four, came to see me with one of the most unusual requests I've encountered. An executive with a large corporation, Evan was despondent because his physical ailment was having a detrimental effect on his marriage, and he wanted me to quickly diagnose and treat his problem—and save his marriage!

His problem started about a year prior to his office visit. While standing, he had increasing pain in his right knee, which was relieved when he sat down. A number of physicians had examined his knee, but no abnormality appeared on X rays and MRI scans of his knee. Physical therapy and knee braces for support had no effect.

So how were his knee problems relevant to his marriage? Not only did Evan work hard, he played hard, too, and he played squash three times a week without any significant pain in his knee. But if his wife wanted to dance with him, his turn on the dance floor lasted only three or four minutes because of pain in his knee. Naturally, his wife didn't understand how he could play squash for hours on end but could not dance for more than four minutes. She suspected an affair! Evan assured me that he loved his wife and was not fooling around.

The answer to the executive's problem showed up in his history. When he played squash, he was bent forward, a position that relieves spinal stenosis. When he was dancing, he was standing, an extended posture that increases the symptoms of spinal stenosis. When I examined him, his knee was normal, but when I asked him to stand in an extended posture for a few minutes, his knee pain returned, and when he sat down, his knee pain resolved. But an MRI of his lumbar spine revealed spinal stenosis, and a course of NSAIDs and epidural corticosteroid injections improved his condition. Soon, Evan was able to play squash and dance with his wife. He believed his diagnosis saved his marriage.

Evan's case is an example of a situation in which physical examination does not reveal a problem unless you exercise until the symptoms appear. At that time sensory, muscle, and reflex changes may become abnormal, but these abnormal findings reverse when back and leg pain resolve. Plain X rays of the lumbar spine may demonstrate degenerative disc disease with facet joint narrowing, but they may not explain the symptoms you experience. MRI scans can be helpful in identifying the location of nerve impingement. CT scans are even better than MRIs at visualizing the bony changes associated with spinal stenosis.

Regardless of test results, the correlation between symptoms and anatomic changes is not as closely associated in spinal stenosis as it is with herniated discs. This has important implications for the role of surgery in the treatment of spinal stenosis.

## Spinal Stenosis: Treatment without Surgery

Treatment of spinal stenosis (neurogenic claudication) starts with becoming educated about the mechanics of the spine and the way your symptoms increase and decrease with this condition. You will understand why you like to bend over the shopping cart in the supermarket and avoid leg pain. Symptoms of spinal stenosis are improved if you sit down, but you can't sit all the time. This is where drug therapy comes in, because it can help improve function.

NSAIDs help treat the pain of osteoarthritis, which is the major cause of spinal stenosis, and these medications are able to decrease swelling in the facet joints as well as the soft tissues in the spinal canal, but there is risk of stomach ulcers. COX-2 inhibitors may be particularly helpful to older osteoarthritis patients who are at risk of developing ulcers. (See chapter 9 for more on these medications.)

Epidural corticosteroid injections may be helpful for leg pain associated with spinal stenosis. However, the sequence of injections is different for spinal stenosis than for herniated disc because the underlying abnormalities are different. With a herniated disc, the acute inflammatory response acts on soft tissues (the gel in the disc) that are herniated. The inflammatory reaction can remove the herniated portion of the disc. At the same time, the inflammatory response irritates the spinal nerve. In order to control the inflammation immediately, epidurals are given as three injections in a short period of time.

I call sixty-eight-year-old Betty "the woman who rode around the world on her bike." Betty had significant spinal stenosis at multiple levels, and an orthopedic surgeon had said that a multilevel operation would be necessary to open the levels that were compressing her nerves and causing leg pain that limited her walking to about two blocks. Betty did not want surgery because she was unsure which level was the most important in controlling her pain. Instead, she chose to have epidural corticosteroid injections when her symptoms required. This meant an injection every four to six months for about twelve years. When she didn't have the injections, she again had difficulty walking two blocks, but with the injections she could get to her health club for regular workouts. Although limited in the standing position, she was quite functional in the seated position, so she rode on a stationary bicycle at least four days a week on a regular basis. Her particular health club counted up her miles, and once she passed the 25,000 mile mark, she was given an "around the world" award, and naturally she wanted to show it to me.

You will be unable to have injections if you are taking blood thinners for clotted blood vessels or artificial heart valve difficulties. Low doses of prednisone rather than epidural injections may work. In older people, corticosteroids are more toxic and should be used only if the drug has a significant beneficial effect on function. If older people are able to get around and are not forced into social isolation because of back and leg pain, the risk-benefit ratio of low-dose corticosteroids favors the drug.

## Weight Loss Works

Questions remain concerning the relationship of obesity and the development of low back pain. Most individuals who are obese do not have back pain. However, back pain that develops when you are overweight can be more resistant to treatment. Movement is an important part of resolving back pain. Getting motivated to move is hard enough when you are in pain, but can be doubly difficult when you are overweight.

Many patients promise that they will lose weight equivalent to an entire arm or leg. A more reasonable goal is two pounds per month. In most circumstances weight loss is part of the therapy to relieve back pain. On occasion it is the therapy to cure back pain.

Diedre is a fifty-four-year-old woman who cured her problem through a thirty-pound weight loss and saved herself an operation. Epidural lipomatosis is an unusual cause of spinal stenosis. Fat is deposited inside the spinal canal and crowds out the spinal nerves. Individuals who are at risk for this problem are those who are obese or require large doses of corticosteroid therapy. Diedre weighed 180 pounds when she presented with persistent low back and leg pain when she walked short distances with an MRI scan demonstrating epidural lipomatosis at two lower lumbar levels. Her choice for therapy was either a potentially dangerous operation to remove all the fat in her canal or to lose weight. There was no guarantee that she would remove the fat from her spine if she lost weight overall, but she was willing to make the effort. Over the next nine months, she was pleased to report to me that her back and leg pain resolved as she lost thirty pounds. She had saved herself an operation and was happy that her weight loss had worked.

## Spinal Stenosis: Indications for Surgery

When pain constantly interferes with walking or leg pain occurs immediately with standing, surgery to remove the stenosis is appropriate. If a single level of stenosis is present and correlates with the reported symptoms, surgical outcome tends to be good. Greater difficulty occurs when multiple levels of stenosis are present and clinical symptoms are diffuse throughout the leg. In these circumstances, an experienced surgeon can complete an appropriate preoperative evaluation to determine the extent of lumbar spine surgery that is required to improve leg pain (see chapter 12).

## SCOLIOSIS

Scoliosis is a lateral curvature of the spine that forms an "S" shape (see fig. 2.1, page 24), the cause of which is unknown in most cases. The spine may also twist like a corkscrew (rotatory scoliosis). Minor curvatures of the spine are common and usually aren't associated with pain or dysfunction.

Although adults get it, scoliosis is most often associated with teenage girls, and some schools now sponsor screening programs that identify at-risk teenagers at an early stage of curvature. Several factors suggest an early scoliosis is developing: one shoulder higher than another, an uneven hemline, the prominence of one shoulder blade compared to the other. When scoliosis is detected early, exercise and a brace may help to avoid surgery later in life. Adults, primarily women, may develop the condition between ages twenty and forty. Most curvatures are stable and do not progress with age. In older people spinal curvature may develop when disc spaces narrow and spinal joints deform.

When younger people develop severe curvatures (over forty degrees), slow spontaneous progression of the deformity results. The imbalance in the spine may also be related to leg length inequalities, when one leg is shorter than the other. However, many such differences are of little consequence, and we don't yet know what degree of difference in leg length is linked with low back pain. A heel lift under the short leg is beneficial in some cases. Progressive curvature has consequences, and vital organs in the chest and abdomen may be squeezed.

Noncritical curvatures are treated with exercises and medications. Young people with severe scoliosis require the placement of metal rods that lengthen the spine and reduce the curvature. Only experienced surgeons should do this operation.

### The Mother with Rods

Sonja complained of increasing low back pain after sitting for long periods at her computer. Now forty-five, she had had scoliosis as a teenager, and because bracing had not worked and the spinal curve was severe, Harrington rods were placed in her spine. She had given birth to two children without difficulty, but now her work required long stints at the computer. She was concerned that her curve was getting worse and her rods were wearing out.

When I examined Sonja, I found that her curve was no worse than it was at the time the rods were first placed. However, the pressure of the rods themselves can place more pressure on the discs and joints of the vertebrae where the clips attach to the spine. She had developed some arthritis at these sites, and range of motion exercises were needed, along with daily nonsteroidal medication. She also joined an aquaerobics (water exercise) program and she swims three times a week. This combination therapy allows her to live normally and do her computer work with minimal discomfort.

Sonja's story helps dispel the misconception that having scoliosis surgery means limited motion and a limited life. In fact, most scoliosis patients can lead normal lives, including having children if they choose, as long as their problem is identified in a timely manner.

---

## DR. B'S PRESCRIPTION SUMMARY

- Back strain is a muscle injury of the low back. Keep moving as much as you can tolerate.
- Disc narrowing is part of the natural aging process that can cause back pain. Flexion (bending forward) exercises help decrease pain and keep you moving.
- Arthritis in your hip can cause pain that is located in your lower back.
- Disc herniations cause back and leg pain made worse with sitting. Sciatica can resolve with extension exercises (bending backward) and oral or injected medications. Disc surgery is required for muscle weakness or intractable pain.
- Spinal stenosis (neurogenic claudication) causes leg pain made worse with walking or standing. Nonsurgical therapy helps the ability to walk longer distances. Surgery improves the condition but does not keep the problem from returning.
- Vascular claudication is leg pain associated with walking that resolves with standing in one place.
- When the "S" curve of scoliosis is severe, it can cause back pain.

---

Chapter 6

# Recognizing and Treating
# Medical Causes of Low Back Pain

MANY MEDICAL ILLNESSES can cause low back pain. Diabetics with nerve damage, for example, feel pain in their back as well as other areas. An undetected bone tumor or cancer can be the cause of back pain. So can problems in nearby organs such as the kidneys or gastrointestinal system. In general, low back pain from a medical condition progresses slowly and persists despite the basic care program. You will also have one of the red flag symptoms mentioned in chapter 1, such as fever or weight loss. It's important that you and your doctor treat the underlying illness, not just the back pain.

## INFECTION

Persistent fever and/or weight loss that accompanies back pain can be infection or a tumor of the spine. Bacterial infections may affect the bone (osteomyelitis), disc (**discitis**), or joint (septic arthritis). The source of the bacteria may be an infection in the skin, urinary tract, oral cavity, or any penetrating wound. Between 1 and 2 percent of people undergoing spinal surgery develop an infection at the surgical site. Some are at increased risk for infections. Diabetics may have decreased immunity to infection because of low antibody levels, as do AIDS (acquired immunodeficiency syndrome) patients. Drug users may use unsterile needles, which allow bacteria to enter the bloodstream, and these bacteria may migrate to the spine and cause pain.

Pain caused by an infection progresses slowly but becomes severe. It is present during rest and made worse by movement. An infection is diagnosed by taking a culture of the organism, either from drawn blood or from the infected area in the spine, which requires placing a needle into the area of infection. Once the organism is identified, the infection is treated with specific antibiotics that will kill the bacteria. It may be necessary to drain the area that acts like an abscess if antibiotics alone are insufficient. The longer it takes to detect the infection, the more likely it is that surgical drainage will be necessary.

## BONE TUMORS AND CANCER

Cancer that involves the lumbar spine can cause loss of appetite and weight loss even before back pain begins. Once pain appears, however, it generally progresses rapidly. Cancers affecting the lumbar spine usually originate in other organs, such as the prostate in men and the breast in women. Multiple myeloma, a bone marrow cancer, is the most common cancer originating in the spinal tissues.

Blood tests may indicate the presence of a tumor. Plain X rays may not identify the location of the tumor, and a bone scan, a test using a small amount of radioactive fluid that is absorbed by inflamed bone, is a sensitive but nonspecific test for identifying bone lesions. MRI and CT scans best identify bony and soft tissue tumor involvement. When a tumor is diagnosed, a biopsy or total removal of the tumor is done, depending on the type, location, and size.

Bone tumors—benign or malignant—of the spinal column or spinal cord are the primary concern in people who have pain at night or when lying flat. Pain results when an expanding tumor and associated inflammation compress the spinal nerves. Although we don't know why, some benign tumors of the spine are more painful at night than during the day.

MRI is the most sensitive method to detect bony abnormalities, spinal cord compression, and soft tissue involvement of tumor-like (malignant) lesions. The abnormal tissue is examined under the microscope to determine if it is benign or cancerous. Therapy depends on the outcome of the diagnostic evaluation. Total removal of the tumor is always preferred as long as vital tissues are not sacrificed.

### "Sleepless" Traveling Salesman

Dennis, a twenty-four-year-old salesperson, thought at first that his yearlong nighttime back pain was related to the fact that he slept in a different bed every night while on the road. Eventually he realized that the beds were not the problem. Dennis's pain increased at night, but aspirin significantly diminished it when he was at home in his own bed. Once he stopped taking aspirin the pain came back.

Plain X rays of his spine showed a "hole" in the L3 vertebra. A bone scan was "hot" (increased bone activity) over the same area without any additional areas of involvement in the remainder of the skeleton. A CT scan identified the exact location of the lesion, and because Dennis was tired of taking aspirin on a daily basis, he had the lesion removed. It was an osteoid osteoma, a benign bone tumor, so its removal was all that was required to eliminate Dennis's back pain.

## INFLAMMATORY DISEASES

Illnesses associated with ongoing inflammation result in disorders that are destructive to spinal tissues. These inflammatory conditions are the result of our immunity losing control. Usually, our immune system fights the "outside world" of bacteria and foreign materials. Our body is able to recognize itself and causes no damage. An abnormal immune system is unable to identify itself. In these circumstances our own immune cells cause damage to our tissues.

### Spinal Inflammatory Arthritis

If morning back stiffness lasts an hour or less, it is probably caused by a mechanical disorder. When it lasts several hours, it would indicate inflammatory arthritis of the spine, or spondyloarthropathy. Inflammatory arthritis of the spine causes the proteins and white cells that fight infection in the bloodstream to attack spinal structures. The lining of the joints, the synovium, swells and impedes motion. With spondyloarthropathies, the body responds to inflammation by depositing calcium in the inflamed tissues. The end result is a spine that has fused facet joints and calcified ligaments.

Rheumatoid arthritis (RA) is a common inflammatory arthritis, but it does not affect the lumbar spine. RA affects most joints in the arms and legs and the cervical spine (neck), but for reasons not yet understood, it spares the lower portion of the spine.

Psoriatic arthritis does cause back pain. Up to 7 percent of people with psoriasis, a common skin disease, also develop this form of arthritis. Most have the skin lesions either prior to or at the same time that the arthritis appears, although a small number have characteristic arthritis symptoms but no evidence of skin abnormalities. Arthritis may be present for ten to twenty years before the psoriatic skin lesions appear.

These conditions and others such as **ankylosing spondylitis** (AS), **reactive arthritis**, and inflammatory bowel disease (IBD) arthritis cause inflammation of the spine (spondylitis).

AS and reactive arthritis are more frequent in men, while psoriatic and IBD spondylitis occur with equal frequency in men and women. AS occurs in 1 percent of the U.S. population; reactive arthritis is the most common cause of arthritis in young adult men. Psoriatic arthritis occurs in 0.1 percent of the general population.

Bilateral sacroiliac joint pain is associated with AS and IBD arthritis and is the initial location for joint inflammation. Reactive arthritis and psoriatic spondylitis may have unilateral sacroiliac joint pain and stiffness or may affect the lumbar spine without involving the sacroiliac joints. AS may affect only the sacroiliac joints or may extend through the entire length of the spine to the cervical spine. AS is not a disease only of joints but is frequently accompanied with severe eye inflammation (iritis), which can lead to blindness if left untreated. In a very few AS patients, the aortic valve of the heart may become leaky and require replacement. IBD arthritis occurs in people with ulcerative colitis and Crohn's disease. The spondyloarthropathy in these patients has similar characteristics to that of AS.

Symptoms of reactive arthritis include superficial eye inflammation (**conjunctivitis**), inflammation of the urinary tract (**urethritis**), and arthritis affecting the spine and lower extremity joints. Reactive arthritis may also include fever, weight loss, and afternoon fatigue. A characteristic skin rash affects the palms and soles and also the tip of the penis. Painless oral ulcers also occur in a few people with reactive arthritis. Occasionally victims of salmonella and shigella epidemics (usually occurring in restaurants and fast food chains) will develop reactive arthritis.

Chlamydia trachomatis, an organism infecting the urinary tract, is linked with the onset of reactive arthritis. (Chlamydia infection is a sexually transmitted disease.) Reactive arthritis patients may develop the whole syndrome of symptoms and signs, including gastrointestinal and urinary symptoms, even if the initial infection occurred in another organ system.

## The Unfortunate Conventioneer

Sidney, thirty, was attending a business convention in the Far East and had unprotected sex with a woman he knew, but whom he had not seen for a number of years. After returning home, he developed fever, gastrointestinal symptoms including diarrhea, and mild pain over his heel. (Heel pain is inflammation of the attachment of tendons to bone, a common location for reactive arthritis inflammation.) Over the next two weeks, Sidney had an episode of conjunctivitis and increasing knee pain. When his primary doctor saw him, Sidney did not mention his sexual encounter or any urinary symptoms, and an evaluation for a gastrointestinal disorder was negative. Only after he developed pain with urination and a rash on his penis did the possibility of reactive arthritis arise. Sidney developed most of the symptoms of the disorder over the next three months.

Sidney's diagnosis was genitourinary chlamydia infection, and he was treated with a course of antibiotics and a COX-2 inhibitor because of a past history of stomach ulcers that increased his risk of bleeding when taking aspirin. After six weeks, all his symptoms except his knee pain were gone, and Sidney still takes a COX-2 inhibitor to control his knee pain.

Sidney's case illustrates the confusion that can arise when the source of the initial infection is overlooked. Always be truthful with your physician about your entire history, including your sexual history. Sidney also illustrates one of the consequences of having unprotected sex. It is entirely possible that Sidney's partner did not know she carried the chlamydia infection, because it may not produce overt symptoms.

## Finding Spondyloarthropathy

Spondyloarthropathy causes stiffness in all directions of spinal motion and tenderness over inflamed portions of the spine. X rays of the lumbosacral spine help to identify early changes of the arthritis, including loss of lumbar curve (lordosis), erosion in the sacroiliac joints, and squaring of vertebral bodies. The front of the vertebral body has an indentation running from the top to the bottom. When a vertebral body is squared, inflammation erodes the prominent part of the top and bottom of the curve. The vertebral body becomes a square.

We do not need to use the more costly radiographic tests to identify the skeletal abnormalities of spondylitis. Histocompatibility testing, a blood test, identifies genetic factors that predispose people to develop spondyloarthropathy. HLA-B27 is a marker associated with these illnesses but does not by itself cause the illness. Approximately 8 percent of the Caucasian U.S. population is B27 positive and does not have a spondyloarthropathy. A total of 7 percent of all HLA-B27 positive Caucasians have AS.

## Therapy of Spine Inflammation

Treatment for the spondyloarthropathies includes range of motion and deep breathing exercises; NSAIDs decrease inflammation and facilitate motion but do not cure the disease. NSAIDs when taken continuously can be helpful in slowing calcification of the spine. Antibiotic therapy for reactive arthritis is most useful early in the course of the illness. Topical therapy for psoriatic skin disease may have a beneficial effect on joint inflammation. Control of IBD may also prove beneficial for joint symptoms.

## Biologic Therapies

A major advance in the treatment of inflammatory arthritis of the spine is the availability of biologic medicines for control of disordered immune function. Biologic therapies consist of antibodies that control increased levels of immune chemicals that cause the inflammatory conditions of the spine. Tumor necrosis factor (TNF) is an immune chemical that is found at increased levels in patients with spondyloarthropathy. Decreasing these levels with the use of anti-TNF therapies is associated with a normalization of immune dysfunction. Some of these anti-TNF therapies used in spondyloarthropathies include etanercept, adalimumab, infliximab, and golimumab.

## Anti-inflammatory Diets

My patients often ask me if diet has any effect on their low back pain. Only about 10 percent of low back pain is caused by an inflammatory disorder like arthritis, and diets that may decrease inflammation have the potential to help the small number with chronic inflammatory lumbar spine conditions.

Fasting diets affect immune function that mediates inflammatory disorders, but this is highly variable and controversial. Fasting for certain periods of time may decrease inflammatory disorders like rheumatoid arthritis through a mechanism of malnutrition that suppresses the body's defense mechanisms. However, the stress of fasting may actually stimulate the immune system. Immune status is also affected by the extent of the fast, whether it is a total or partial fast. In any case, fasting must be closely monitored.

Food sensitivities can also stimulate the immune response. The gastrointestinal tract in people who develop arthritis may allow certain foods that usually would not be absorbed, such as the proteins in cow's milk, to enter the body. When this happens, the body responds by producing antibodies to signal increased immune response that may be associated with joint, muscle, or blood vessel inflammation. Experimentation with elimination diets has suggested that removing eggs, milk, chocolate, wheat, beans, and shellfish from the diet may be helpful.

Vegetarian diets, supplemented with nuts, eggs, and dairy products (unless sensitivities to these foods are present), along with antioxidants and B vitamins, may also decrease joint inflammation. In general, reducing animal fats in the diet and taking antioxidant supplements may decrease the level of inflammation.

### Fatty Acid Supplements

Eliminating foods from the diet to control pain and inflammation may not be as helpful as adding certain foods. For example, consuming cold-water fish such as salmon and mackerel may help decrease inflammation. The connection between fish and inflammation has to do with the fats in the membranes of our cells. These membrane fats are the sources of the chemicals that produce prostaglandins (PG), which are one of the factors that promote inflammation and pain. Fish oils, specifically the omega-3 family of polyunsaturated fatty acids (EPA, DHA), are different from human oils (arachidonic acid). The prostaglandins formed with fish oils are less inflammatory than those formed with arachidonic acid. When you consume cold-water fish, you can replace the fats in the membranes of your cells with fish oils. This in turn results in less inflammation and pain.

Any of these diets takes time to work. In addition, it is necessary to implement a significant substitution before anti-inflammatory effects occur. Fish oil supplements may hasten this substitution, but amounts of three to five grams per day may be necessary to obtain the beneficial effect. You may need to consume so much omega-3 fatty acid that you may start taking on a fishy aroma.

Plant sources of special fatty acids such as gamma linolenic acid (GLA) include flaxseed, evening primrose, and borage oils. These sources of fatty acids also produce prostaglandins that are less inflammatory. A significant amount of these plant oils are needed on a daily basis to achieve an anti-inflammatory effect. The problem with some of these plant and fish fatty acids is that they contain calories. A consultation with a physician or nutritionist would result in a diet that includes these fatty acids while maintaining a reasonable daily calorie intake.

### Bread-free Diets

Another form of diet that may help relieve back pain involves the elimination of wheat from your diet. Celiac disease is a disorder associated with sensitivity to gluten, the protein in wheat, barley, and rye. Individuals with this sensitivity have malabsorption associated with bloating, diarrhea, and nutritional deficiencies including vitamins. On occasion, back pain can be part of the symptoms associated with this disorder, possibly related to the lack of vitamins. My "bread-free patient" taught me this lesson. She had an intermittent complaint of back pain that did not follow any particular pattern. She could have pain day or night that would come and go. She had some difficulty with bowel symptoms when she would eat bread but did not associate the event with her back pain. She decided to eliminate bread from her diet and within a few weeks her back pain resolved. She told me, given the choice, she will get the gluten-free bread to keep from getting back pain again.

## DISH SYNDROME (DIFFUSE IDIOPATHIC SKELETAL HYPEROSTOSIS)

DISH syndrome affects the spine and is sometimes confused with AS. It is different from AS because the sacroiliac joints are unaffected while the front of the spine is altered, leaving the facet joints untouched. The two disorders are often confused because DISH, like AS, causes calcification of the spine. DISH occurs most commonly in Caucasian men fifty and older, compared to AS, which often affects people in their twenties. DISH may be asymptomatic and often is detected only on X rays.

Morning stiffness and decreased range of motion usually lasts an hour or less, and back pain is higher in the spine near the thorax. No organ systems other than the bone and joints are affected, and HLA-B27 is negative in DISH patients. X rays of the spine show flowing calcifications (resembling candle wax) on the anterior portion of at least four thoracic vertebrae. The lumbar spine is affected less frequently.

Treatment for DISH involves movement (strongly recommended) and deep breathing exercises. No therapy exists that removes the calcifications in the spine, and surgical removal is not appropriate.

## OCHRONOSIS

This is another rare and unusual illness that may be confused with AS. Ochronosis is caused by the accumulation of a chemical, homogentisic acid, in tissues. Over time, this accumulated chemical becomes black, and the deposits blacken many areas, including the ears and the whites of the eyes. The chemical is also passed in the urine, thereby making it black if it is exposed to the sun. The same chemical settles in the tissues around the spine and causes calcifications that mimic AS. No effective therapy exists. Fortunately, ochronosis is extremely rare, occurring in about 1 in 10 million people.

## FIBROMYALGIA

Fibromyalgia (FM) is a soft tissue pain syndrome characterized by chronic pain in discrete tender point areas, including the lumbar spine; but it is not associated with any structural abnormalities of muscle, bone, or cartilage. The persistent pain and chronic fatigue associated with the illness prevent those who have it from achieving their full potential. It also brings with it tension headaches, irritable bowel syndrome, and low blood pressure.

Although controversy exists about the existence of FM, about 15 percent of people who visit a rheumatologist satisfy the criteria for this disorder. Women, particularly young and middle-aged women, are affected more frequently than men. In about half the cases, the onset of FM seems to follow an injury, excessive physical activity, or emotional or psychological stress. The pain may be unremitting with durations of up to twenty years, or the discomfort may be migratory and wax and wane.

Fatigue is also a prominent feature of FM, and these patients often report restless sleep and morning exhaustion. Cold or humid weather, overactivity, total inactivity, stress, menses, and poor sleep exacerbate FM. Symptoms improve with moderate activity; warm, dry weather; and massage.

Areas that are tender to palpation are referred to as tender points and are localized, most commonly to the upper border of the shoulders, knees, elbows, and the lumbar spine. There is no pain outside the area. There may be twelve or more sensitive areas in someone with primary FM. Other than identifying these tender points, a physical examination usually is normal. The diagnosis of FM is based on eliminating other conditions.

The American College of Rheumatology in 1990 reported classification criteria for FM that includes a history of widespread pain for a minimum of three months (pain in four body quadrants) and pain in eleven of eighteen tender points when manually palpated. In addition, the presence of another disorder does not exclude a diagnosis of FM. Updated versions of the criteria do not concentrate on the presence of tender points as much as the presence of generalized widespread pain. In a study involving patients who'd had spinal surgery and who were referred to a spine center for lumbar pain, 12 percent had FM complicating their condition, but the FM had remained undiagnosed.

Treatment of FM requires a multifaceted approach. In many circumstances, educating the patients about their illness is reassuring and relieves some symptoms. Most people are encouraged to know their symptoms are not "all in their head." Once they understand that their condition is not life threatening, deforming, or degenerating, even though it causes chronic pain, they can adjust their lifestyle.

Rest and relaxation are important for FM patients who are overworked. You are generally encouraged to remain at work if possible, while at the same time avoiding excessive fatigue. Range of motion and stretching exercises encourage improved muscle function, and an aerobic exercise program is also essential. Heat treatments are also useful.

NSAIDs help reduce FM-related pain. Tramadol (Ultram), a nonopioid analgesic, also may be helpful. The new drug combination of tramadol and acetaminophen (Ultracet) provides enhanced pain relief compared to the individual components of the drug. Long-acting forms of tramadol taken once a day have the benefit of a sustained analgesic effect. To control localized pain, tender points can be injected with a combination of anesthetic agent and a long-acting corticosteroid.

Antidepressants such as the tricyclic Elavil (amitriptyline) and muscle relaxants like Flexeril (cyclobenzaprine) increase the brain's serotonin to influence mood. Increased levels of serotonin reduce pain and induce sleep. Other antidepressant therapies, such as duloxetine and milnacipran, have been approved for the treatment of FM. Drugs called selective serotonin reuptake inhibitors (SSRIs) like Prozac (fluoxetine) or Zoloft (sertraline) may help certain people, but in general, this class of antidepressants does not work as effectively for FM as the tricyclic drugs.

A type of antiseizure drug is another category of medicine that is effective for the treatment of FM. Lyrica (pregablin) is an example of this category of drug for FM.

The basic therapeutic program for FM involves patient education, aerobic exercise, and a medication (pregabalin or cyclobenzaprine). Adding an NSAID is optional and depends on the patient's muscle pain. Injecting tender points is useful if they are few in number. Over the long term, compliance with the program is essential.

## POLYMYALGIA RHEUMATICA

Polymyalgia rheumatica (PMR) is a clinical syndrome characterized by severe stiffness, tenderness, and aching of the muscles around the buttocks and shoulders. If you are sixty years or older, you are more at risk for this disorder. The majority of individuals with PMR have the sudden onset of severe muscle pain that is particularly worse in the mornings and after being sedentary for even short periods of time. Getting out of bed can be particularly difficult. You may also develop fatigue, weight loss, and fever.

Patients with PMR have tenderness on palpation of the muscles around the low back, buttocks, and thighs. The muscles around the shoulders and neck are also tender. The movement of the hips, back, neck, and shoulders may be limited because of muscle pain.

Blood tests are abnormal in PMR patients. The vast majority will have an elevated erythrocyte sedimentation rate and/or C-reactive protein level. Low-grade anemia is another common abnormality.

Treatment of PMR is an adequate dose of corticosteroids, like prednisone, that relieves muscle pain and lowers the elevated erythrocyte sedimentation rate (ESR) levels. The response to therapy is monitored by repeating ESR tests. About a third of patients are better in about one year; another third are better in up to two years, and a third need persistent prednisone therapy at low doses. The majority of PMR patients have resolution of low back pain with appropriate therapy.

## TENSION MYOSITIS SYNDROME

Generalized muscle tension in people with chronic anxiety and stress causes pain, and this phenomenon has been given a name: tension myositis syndrome (TMS). Dr. John Sarno, who popularized the TMS diagnosis, suggests that the autonomic nervous system, in response to repressed emotions like anxiety and anger, causes a decrease of blood flow to muscles, which results in oxygen deprivation, known as ischemia.

According to Dr. Sarno's proposition, ischemia is the reason for pain in muscles, tendons, and ligaments. Muscle tension is also thought to occur in a similar manner in FM. In this way, Sarno proposes that TMS and FM are similar disorders and treatment is psychological, not physical. If the repressed thoughts are removed, the pain will resolve.

Although I believe that the central nervous system plays a significant role in the response to pain, I do not agree with the hypothesis upon which TMS is based. I have had a number of patients with back strain or fibromyalgia who have not had any increase in muscle tension although they have been exquisitely sensitive at tender points, many of which are over ligaments or tendons, not muscles. In addition, when compared to muscles, ligaments and tendons require minimal amounts of oxygen to function. Ischemia would have a significantly different effect on these tissues.

Undoubtedly, chronic pain can make you anxious, but being anxious does not cause low back pain, which can be modified by changes in physical positions. As for therapy, I would agree with Dr. Sarno that physical activity is beneficial in restoring function. Resolving stressful issues is good for everyone, those with low back pain and those without it. To control chronic pain it is necessary to reduce anxiety and reverse fatigue. But, if you have AS (inflammation of the spine) for example, you can't expect your pain to go away just because you resolve your anger with your boss, or you change jobs, or you work through other stressful problems.

## MYOFASCIAL PAIN SYNDROME

Low back pain is a common symptom of myofascial pain syndrome (MPS). Remember the fascia is that "plastic wrap" covering of your muscles. MPS is a regional pain syndrome with two major symptoms: a localized area of deep muscle tenderness (trigger point) accompanied by a palpable nodule in the muscle, and a specific area of referred pain distant from the trigger point.

Pressure over a trigger point creates a dull, aching pain in a referral pattern that does not follow any characteristic muscle structure. Although the symptoms may sound similar, FM and MPS are not the same illness. MPS is a localized pain syndrome with sudden onset and trigger points that radiate pain. Treatment for MPS involves injecting trigger points with anesthetics, along with the use of superficial cooling and muscle stretching.

## BLOOD AND VESSEL DISORDERS

Hemoglobin is the protein that carries oxygen to our tissues, and if the proteins making up hemoglobin develop abnormalities, their ability to carry oxygen to tissues is compromised. Red blood cells also may change shape, which then impedes flow in the small blood vessels. Hemoglobinopathies are a group of blood disorders that cause abnormalities of the hemoglobin that packs the red cells in our blood. The primary example is sickle cell anemia. When oxygen levels are low, red blood cells will lose their normal shape and become sickled. Sickled cells will clog small blood vessels throughout the body, which is part of what we call a sickle cell crisis. The spinal vertebrae are primary locations for this blood vessel change. Lack of oxygen causes death of tissues, in this case, bone tissue. Bone death (avascular necrosis) is readily apparent on X rays of the lumbar spine.

No therapy currently is available to reverse the single amino acid substitution that results in the abnormal hemoglobin. In the future, the ability to substitute normal genetic code for abnormal codes will offer the cure for this illness. Until that time, sickle cell patients are treated with intravenous fluids, pain medications, and oxygen.

### Aneurysms

Throbbing pain may occur in your low back with an aneurysm of the abdominal aorta. The aorta is the major arterial blood vessel that supplies blood from the heart to the rest of the body and runs just in front of the lumbar spine. An aneurysm is a weakening in the wall of the vessel, and is analogous to weakening in the sidewall of a tire. As the tire weakens, the remaining wall experiences increasing pressure. If the pressure becomes too great, the tire may blow out. Similarly, if the pressure on the wall of the vessel occurs, then an aneurysm will rupture.

There may be no symptoms with a slowly growing aneurysm, but vascular changes may be noted on X rays of the abdomen taken for other reasons. Pain frequently increases as the aneurysm grows. Abdominal aneurysms occur most commonly in Caucasian men between ages sixty and seventy. Individuals at high risk for aneurysms have high cholesterol levels, many years of heavy smoking, high blood pressure, and/or a family history of aneurysm.

Physical examination of the abdomen reveals a pulsating mass. X rays reveal the aneurysm if there is calcification in the vessel wall, and a CT scan is very good at identifying the extent and size of the lesions. Injecting intravenous dye to better determine the arteries included in the aneurysm is a procedure usually reserved for those who are candidates for surgery. Aneurysms of five centimeters or less can be watched, but those six centimeters or more require bypass surgery. This elective procedure is associated with 2 percent mortality, but the mortality rises to 30 percent once the vessel has ruptured.

### DIABETIC NEUROPATHY

If glucose (sugar) levels get too high in the bloodstream of a diabetic for a long period of time, peripheral nerves that supply signals for sensation and muscle function are damaged. One of these nerves, the femoral, runs down the front of the thigh. Diabetes can cause a femoral neuropathy, which causes pain and weakness in the thigh.

Pain from peripheral neuropathy does not change with position, and this tells us it is not the kind of radicular pain we see with a disc herniation. The symptoms related to diabetes are improved when glucose levels return to normal, which is usually accomplished with oral medications or insulin injections. An internist or endocrinologist can help you with the therapies necessary to control diabetes.

### PAIN FROM NEARBY ORGANS

Abnormalities in organs that share nerves with part of the spine can cause referred back pain. It can arise from gastrointestinal, vascular, or genitourinary disorders. The duration and sequence of back pain follows the characteristics of the diseased organ. For example, colicky pain is characterized by repeated spasms of intense pain followed by pain-free periods. This kind of pain is associated with spasm in a hollow structure such as the ureter, colon, or gallbladder.

Anyone who has had a kidney stone understands severe colicky pain. Kidney and gallbladder pain occur in the upper portion of the lumbar spine while colonic pain occurs lower, near the sacrum. Abnormalities in these organ systems appear as blood in the urine or stool, or increasing pain when fatty foods are consumed. After eating spicy foods, individuals with ulcers in the stomach or small intestine may experience pain in the midline of the upper lumbar spine. It can often be quite difficult to determine the causes of the different types of back pain, and the job is made more difficult, of course, because the same person can experience pain from more than one cause.

### Retroperitoneal Disorders

The retroperitoneum is the area in front of the lumbar spine. Any disorder that causes swelling in this area of the back causes pain that radiates from the low back through the front of the abdomen to the anterior thigh. The organs in the retroperitoneum include the kidneys, lymph glands, aorta, and large muscle groups (psoas). Kidney tumors, cancer of the lymph glands, aortic aneurysm, or bleeding into the large muscle groups can cause pain that appears in the anterior thigh, although its origin is in the lumbar spine. An MRI scan of the retroperitoneum will identify most of the organs that cause pain in this distribution.

## BACK PAIN IN PREGNANCY AND MENSTRUATION

Half of all pregnant women develop moderate to severe back pain. This pain can be from hormonal changes that alter the flexibility of ligaments and joints in the pelvis, or simply the mechanical problem of the added weight in the pelvis. The pressure on the supporting structures in the pelvis, or a marked increase in the lumbar curve (lordosis), strains the supporting muscles. In the nonpregnant state there is practically no motion in the joints of the pelvis, the front of the pelvis, and sacroiliac joints. However, during pregnancy, a hormone, relaxin, is produced and it allows increased motion of the pelvic joints, and this causes tension in the relaxed capsule and ligaments. Increased lordosis also increases the weakness of the abdominal muscles and puts greater strain on the muscles near the spine. Active movement such as climbing stairs increases the strain.

Being physically fit before pregnancy may cut your risk of developing back pain. If a pregnancy is in your future, a physical fitness program with aerobic and strengthening exercises is helpful. Exercises and external supports can be helpful to you if you are already pregnant and have back pain,

You can decrease your back pain by lying on your side and by exercising in a swimming pool to strengthen your muscles while limiting strain on the lower extremities.

Acetaminophen (Tylenol) is the only pain medication that is safe during pregnancy. In rare circumstances, if symptoms persist, a new mother may require bracing after delivery.

Most women find that extension exercises (bending backward) are most helpful (see chapter 10). The problem is that after the first three months, most pregnant women are unable to rest on their stomachs to do this. You can do extension exercises while standing by placing your hands on the low back and bending backward. You can lean on a table and bend backward. Kneel on the floor and rest your upper body on a chair and increase the curve in your back.

If you have pain on one side of your back, try lying down on the side with the pain and put a small pillow at your waist.

Supporting your abdomen may also decrease pain. Place your hands under your abdomen and lift gently. If your back pain decreases, you are a candidate for a corset with a flexible band in front that expands as you enlarge through your pregnancy.

The good news is that back pain resolves when the baby is born. Only a very small minority of women continue to have pain months after the pregnancy is concluded.

Back pain that coincides with a woman's menstrual cycle may be related to endometriosis, a disease in which tissue from the lining of the uterus (endometrium) is present outside the uterine cavity. The endometrial tissue may be located on the ovaries or at the bottom of the pelvis near the rectum. Pain is a part of this disease because endometrial tissue outside the uterus undergoes the same monthly cycle of growth, shedding, and bleeding as the tissues inside the uterus. While the disease may occur at any age after the onset of menses, incidence rises as women reach their late twenties or thirties. Overall, just over 3 percent of women of reproductive age develop endometriosis. When the endometriosis involves the colon and ureter, back pain is usually present. Pain increases at the time of menstruation and persists throughout the entire time of bleeding.

Endometriosis may render the abdomen tender over the uterus or ovary or other organs to which the endometrium has attached. Endometriosis is often diagnosed through laparoscopy, a relatively simple surgical procedure that allows us to view the inside of the abdomen. Organ tissue can be biopsied to determine the presence of endometrial tissue.

Endometriosis is usually treated with oral contraceptives or other medications that suppress menstruation, thereby suppressing the growth of the endometrium. Pregnancy will also suppress endometrial growth, but many women with endometriosis have difficulty conceiving because the disease leads to infertility.

## DR. B'S PRESCRIPTION SUMMARY

- Red flags are a sign of more serious systemic illness.
- Fever is associated with a back infection.
- Severe pain while lying down at night is caused by bone tumors.
- Prolonged morning stiffness is a characteristic of inflammatory arthritis of the spine.
- Bone pain is caused by fractures like those associated with osteoporosis.
- Crampy pain comes from other organs like the uterus, intestines, or ureter.
- Generalized muscle pain is caused by FM.
- TMS does not exist.
- Severe muscle pain and stiffness getting out of bed in the morning is associated with PMR.
- Pregnant women can decrease back pain by exercising in a swimming pool to strengthen muscles while limiting strain on the legs, or by lying on their side.

Chapter 7

# How Can I Keep from Getting Bent Over?

AS OUR POPULATION grows older, an increasing number of people will develop back pain. Back pain in older women and men can be from mechanical or systemic disorders. The vast majority have pain related to mechanical problems of the spine (see chapter 5). However, systemic disorders are becoming a greater percentage of back problems as our population ages. A systemic problem associated with fracture of bones in the lumbar spine is osteoporosis. The good news about this problem is that it is preventable. In those people where a fracture occurs, it is treatable.

## OSTEOPOROSIS

Osteoporosis is most common in Caucasian postmenopausal women, but it also affects African American, Asian, and Hispanic women. Men cannot afford to be complacent, because they account for about 20 percent of osteoporosis cases. Ten million Americans have osteoporosis, with another 18 million at risk for fracture because of decreased bone mineral density. The primary locations in the skeleton for osteoporosis include the spine, hip bone, pelvis, and wrist.

Bone is made up of a framework of collagen that is like the girders of a building. A mineral compound containing calcium and phosphorus forms the cement that layers the girders. Just as our soft tissues are alive and always changing, bone is continuously being remodeled by cells that excavate (osteoclasts) and rebuild (osteoblasts). Our bones are a constant source of calcium that is carried by the bloodstream throughout the body. Calcium is an essential element in a number of normal functions, including muscle contraction. During our youth, calcium is absorbed and stored in bone, and the building cells, the osteoblasts, predominate. As we age, the excavating cells, osteoclasts, are more active, which results in calcium loss. If the calcium content becomes too low, the bone is weakened and is at risk for fracture.

The peak bone mass in the spine and hip bones is reached by age eighteen in women. Bone mass remains stable until menopause, when a reduction of estrogen results in a phase of rapid bone loss. Bone loss continues at a slower pace for the following decades. As the calcium is lost from bone, the bone architecture is altered with many of the cross-struts supporting weight being lost. This compromises bone strength and increases fracture risk.

### Risk Factors

Primary risk factors for osteoporosis include female sex, increased age, estrogen deficiency, family history of osteoporosis, white race, low body weight, smoking, and history of fractures. Osteoporosis may also occur as a secondary condition to medical disorders and medications such as long-term use of corticosteroids like prednisone. Normal hormonal changes that occur after menopause are linked with osteoporosis. If fractures have occurred in the thoracic spine, a kyphosis—dowager's hump—may be present. This is an exaggerated forward curve of the thoracic spine that pushes the head and chest forward.

Spinal pain localized in the middle of the back over the bone is associated with disorders that fracture or expand bone. Any systemic process that increases calcium loss from bone (osteoporosis), causes bone death (sickle cell anemia), or replaces bone cells with inflammatory or cancer cells (multiple myeloma) weakens vertebral bone to the point that fracture may occur spontaneously or with minimal trauma. Acute fractures create sudden onset of severe pain, but the pain may be the initial manifestation of the underlying disorder. Most osteoporotic bone is painless until it fractures.

When measured, osteoporotic individuals have lost height. A loss of two inches is an indicator of spinal fractures. Some individuals have lost so much height that the edge of their ribs comes close to their pelvic bones. These individuals have rib pain and shortness of breath

Not all height loss is related to osteoporosis. Some of my patients are amazed that they have lost height but have strong bones. It is important to remember that growing shorter can come from flattening intervertebral discs. This loss of disc height can add up to a significant shortening if enough levels are affected.

### Finding Fractures and Measuring Bone Mineral Density

X rays may show alterations in the bone but do not reveal small fractures. A bone scan can detect increased bone activity soon after a fracture occurs, and a CT scan may identify the abnormality. However, locating the lesion is not enough to allow us to determine the specific cause of the bony changes.

### Fractured Frannie

Frannie is a seventy-two-year-old woman who has risk factors for osteoporosis. She had a fall on her buttocks. She developed pain over the sacrum and **coccydynia.** She had difficulty walking. Plain X rays of the sacrum and coccyx demonstrated no fractures. She had to walk with a cane because of severe low back pain. I evaluated her and found specific areas of pain over the sacrum. An MRI scan was obtained but was read as not having a fracture. I believed that her most likely cause of her pain was a fracture. A CT scan of the pelvis showed a fracture of the sacrum. She was treated with Miacalcin (calcitonin), Fosamax (alendronate), and Ultram (tramadol). Over the following six weeks her coccydynia and sacral pain resolved. She discontinued her Fosamax after ten years of therapy.

Dual energy X ray absorptiometry (DXA) is the method most frequently used to determine bone mineral density in the spine and the thighbone. Low-energy X rays are used to determine the difference in the absorption of the beam by the bone versus the soft tissues. Bone tissue will absorb the beam of X rays, whereas X rays will pass through the soft tissues. The difference in absorption corresponds to the amount of calcium in the bones. The best candidates for this test are postmenopausal women, and men and women taking corticosteroids. This method is the most efficient way of measuring the level of bone mineral in your hip and spine.

The results of the DXA exam are reported as an absolute value of grams/cubic centimeter, and as a comparison to age-race, and sex-matched individuals (Z score), and as a comparison to the average bone mass of young adult normal individuals (T score). A change of 1 standard deviation of a Z or T score correlates with a change of 0.06 g/cm².

Quantitative computed tomography (QCT) uses a larger dose of X ray to determine the true volume of bone mineral. QCT is also able to distinguish different types of bone structure. However, the extra expense and the X ray exposure have limited the common use of this technique for bone mineral density (BMD) measurement.

Ultrasound uses sound waves to determine the bone mineral content of bone. Sound waves are unable to penetrate bone, making a specific determination of bone calcium very difficult. Therefore, ultrasound is an insensitive technique for making the diagnosis of osteoporosis. Individuals with abnormalities on ultrasound tests should have a DXA test.

## OSTEOPOROSIS DIAGNOSIS

Osteoporosis is diagnosed in individuals who experience nontraumatic fractures of the hip, spine, or wrist related to falls from low heights. In fact, some individuals fracture their hip and then fall. In the absence of a fracture, BMD can be used to diagnose osteoporosis. The World Health Organization (WHO) defines osteoporosis as a T score < −2.5 standard deviations below the mean value of peak bone mass. Osteopenia is a BMD T score between −1 and −2.5.

An actual risk of developing a hip or spine fracture over the next ten years is determined by the Fracture Risk Assessment (FRAX) tool. This calculator was developed by the WHO to determine risk without the need for radiographs. The tool is available on the web at www.shef .ac.uk/FRAX. The tool takes into account eleven clinical risk factors and hip BMD, if available, to give the risk of developing fractures.

## MEN AND OSTEOPOROSIS

Osteoporosis is less common in men than women. Men have larger skeletons; bone loss starts later in life and progresses more slowly. Men do not have the rapid loss of bone related to estrogen loss though men do produce low levels of estrogen. Bone loss does occur in men as testosterone levels decrease. The ability to absorb calcium is decreased while the time devoted to exercise declines with age. The risk for fracture also increases with the tendency to fall more often.

Secondary osteoporosis is the form of the illness that occurs related to an illness that affects bone (malabsorption), therapies that decrease bone mineral density (corticosteroids), or unhealthy lifestyle (smoking, excessive alcohol). In men, hormone ablation therapy for prostate cancer can result in an increased risk.

Osteoporosis is as serious a medical condition for men as it is for women. In the year following a hip fracture, up to 20 percent of patients die. Nursing home care is required for another 20 percent, and 50 percent of individuals never fully recover.

## KEEP YOUR BONES STRONG

Starting at an early age, our goal should be to prevent osteoporosis before our bones reach that stage when they weaken and become thin. This means maximizing our bone calcium during adolescence; maintaining bone calcium during adulthood; and for women, minimizing postmenopausal bone loss. Bone calcium increases in children and adolescents who consume higher levels of calcium in food or supplements. However, high calcium intake during the postmenopausal period has no effect—or a minimal protective effect—against bone loss in women.

### Calcium/Vitamin D

To maintain bone strength, most adults should have 1000 to 1500 mg of calcium per day. Calcium should be taken in divided doses with meals. Taking calcium with meals increases the potential of absorption with other nutrients from a meal. Calcium citrate and carbonate are supplement forms of calcium. Citrate is easier to absorb. In addition, regular weight-bearing exercise, like walking, contributes to the development of bone mass, and resistance or impact exercise, such as lifting weights, helps maintain bone mineral levels. You should be sure that your calcium preparation is absorbable. Some house-brand preparations are not.

Frances is a fifty-four-year-old woman who told me that she was taking her oyster-shell calcium on a regular basis. She thought she was absorbing it all. Was she surprised when I showed her the X ray of the lumbar spine that she had taken for back pain. We were able to count seven calcium pills in her lower intestinal tract. If we could count them, they were not being absorbed. I told her to throw out the ones she had, and get a brand-name calcium citrate or carbonate product; I also told her to do a vinegar test.

Not all calcium supplements dissolve in the stomach. Your preparation may be like Frances's that did not dissolve. Take your calcium tablet and place it in a glass filled about one-third with regular vinegar. Swirl the vinegar around and let it sit for about thirty minutes. When you come back the calcium tablet should be dissolving. If not, throw them out. If it will not dissolve in the glass, it will not dissolve in your stomach.

In Caucasian women, calcium intake should be 800 mg a day until age ten, then 1500 mg during adolescence and pregnancy, and 1200 mg during adulthood. Vitamin D, 400 to 800 IU, is a valuable supplement used in conjunction with calcium supplements. This is particularly helpful for the elderly who have limited exposure to sunlight, or nutritional deficiency. Vitamin D levels can be quantified through blood tests. Higher levels of supplementation can be taken if serum levels are inadequate. The combination of these supplements decreases the risk of hip fractures in elderly populations. Non-Caucasian women start with a greater amount of bone mineral calcium. They should take calcium supplements, but they are at less risk for fractures.

## Hormone Replacement Therapy for Women

The reason osteoporosis is considered a women's health issue is because estrogen deficiency after menopause leads to bone loss. The greatest rate of bone loss occurs in the first years after cessation of ovarian function. Estrogen replacement therapy, commonly called ERT, is often started soon after the onset of menopause in women who are appropriate candidates. Some women begin hormonal therapy during the perimenopausal periods. ERT is not recommended if you have a history of breast or uterine cancer or clotting disorders. To prevent bone loss with ERT, women need estrogen every day. For women with an intact uterus, progesterone is added because it decreases the risk of uterine cancer. This combination therapy is called HRT, hormone replacement therapy. The Women's Health Initiative, a large, national study of women taking estrogen and progesterone replacement therapy, reported an increase in cardiovascular disease and breast cancer in the group taking HRT. The study was stopped prematurely because of the concerns regarding the ill effects of HRT. The appropriate role of HRT remains very much in question. The use of HRT is a personal choice that must be discussed with your physician.

Raloxifene (Evista) is a selective estrogen receptor modulator (SERM) with estrogen-like effects on bone resorption but without stimulating breast tissue or the lining of the uterus in postmenopausal women. Raloxifene, given in daily doses, effectively increases bone and decreases the risk of spine and hip fracture. Toxic side effects include hot flashes, leg cramps, and rare episodes of venous clotting.

## Calcitonin

Calcitonin is a hormone that reduces bone breakdown and is used to treat osteoporosis, and salmon calcitonin is more effective than human calcitonin. Calcitonin is given by injection, or intranasally, on a daily basis. Nasal calcitonin decreases the risk of spinal fractures but may not significantly alter the risk of hip fractures. However, one of the added benefits of calcitonin is its pain-relieving effects, particularly on bone fractures.

## Bisphosphonates

**Bisphosphonates** came into medical use in a roundabout way, and their concept is based on research that studied detergents and hard water. Bisphosphonates attach to bone crystals, the sites of active bone remodeling. Bones are living tissues, constantly being built up and torn down, and bisphosphonates alter bone remodeling by reducing the tearing down portion of remodeling. By decreasing bone resorption, bone density is increased.

Alendronate (Fosamax) effectively prevents and treats osteoporosis because alendronate is a potent inhibiting agent of bone remodeling. Studies of women with established osteoporosis have found that alendronate given once a week prevents postmenopausal bone loss and increases bone density in the spine by approximately 4 to 6 percent over a three year period. Alendronate also has a beneficial effect on increasing bone density in the hip. The effect on bone is prolonged, meaning that it's measured in years; therefore, younger women of childbearing years are not candidates for this agent. The weekly dose formulation is more convenient than the smaller daily dose. This weekly regimen decreases exposure of the esophagus and, hence, reduces irritation. Alendronate is available in a generic form.

Risedronate (Actonel) decreases the risk of spine and hip fractures as well as increases bone in these locations. This drug is approved by the Food and Drug Administration (FDA) for the treatment of postmenopausal osteoporosis at a single daily dose. Act-onel as a once-weekly or a once-monthly pill is also available.

Ibandronate (Boniva) is a bisphosphonate that can be taken orally or intravenously. The oral preparation is given once a month. You need to take the pill with a large glass of water first thing in the morning and remain upright without ingesting any food for at a least an hour. This process allows the drug to be alone in the digestive tract, maximiz-ing absorption. Another option for you if you develop gastrointestinal irritation from oral bisphosphonates is the intravenous form of iban-dronate. Ibandronate can be given by vein every three months. The infusion is given by a "push." A push infusion takes about two to three minutes to administer. Side effects from the infusion are no differ-ent that those of the oral form of the medicine as long as the medicine remains in the vein.

Zoledronic acid (Reclast) is a form of bisphosphonate therapy that is solely available as an intravenous medicine. One benefit of this form of therapy is that infusions are only once a year. As opposed to iban-dronate the infusion duration is longer, usually measured in fifteen to thirty minutes.

The primary toxicity of the bisphosphonates is gastrointestinal, and they tend to have poor intestinal absorption. These drugs must be taken on an empty stomach. For example, alendronate should be taken in the morning after an overnight fast, with a large glass of water. In addition, you should remain upright for thirty minutes to assure that the medication remains out of the esophagus, because heartburn is a common complaint.

### How Long Bisphosphonates?

The duration of therapy with alendronate and other bisphosphonates has become an increasingly important question as individuals con-tinue to ingest the medicine for ten years or longer. The concern is that individuals who have consumed bisphosphonates for prolonged periods may be at risk of developing stress fractures in the hip bones. The location of the fractures lower on the thighbone suggests that these breaks are related to therapy and not osteoporosis. These fractures have appeared between five to ten years after starting bisphospho-nates. Studies of large populations have reported conflicting results. At this point there is no conclusive evidence to stop bisphosphonate therapy. However, the benefits of bisphosphonate therapy does diminish over time. What to do?

The patients at risk are those who have consumed bisphosphonates for over five years. A suggestion that should be considered is to stop bisphosphonates and measure BMD with a DXA at a year to determine if the deposition of bisphosphonate in bone over time is adequate to maintain bone strength. You could remain off bisphosphonates if BMD has remained stable. Restarting bisphosphonates or commencing alternative therapy, like teriparatide, should be considered.

### Human Parathyroid Hormone

Parathyroid hormone is a protein that is usually associated with dissolving of bone to maintain blood levels of calcium. Normal levels of calcium are essential for the normal functioning of the muscles, including the heart. Our bones are the storehouse of calcium and parathyroid is the chisel that chips bone away. What we have come to realize through a number of experiments is that when small amounts of parathyroid hormone are injected on a daily basis, an opposite effect happens. The osteoblasts, the cells that build bone, are stimulated. New bone is made when parathyroid hormone is injected in this way.

Teriparatide is indicated for individuals who have already developed bone fractures: by definition, individuals who have vertebral or hip fractures. Bone mass is usually deficient when spontaneous fractures occur. Bone mass is increased more rapidly with parathyroid hormone than bisphosphonates. Therefore, teriparatide is the preferred therapy if more rapid bone mass is required.

Teriparatide (Forteo) is an injectable form of parathyroid hormone. A subcutaneous injection of the thigh or abdomen of 20 mcg daily may be given for up to two years. The medicine is delivered with an auto-injector pen that injects the medicine automatically when the pen is primed when placed on the skin. Toxicities of this medicine include nausea and transient dizziness. The drug is limited to a two-year duration since soft tissue tumors appeared in rats who took higher doses of medicine for longer periods of time.

Joseph is a seventy-year-old man with prostate cancer treated with antitestosterone therapy for over two years. He slipped, falling onto his buttocks. He immediately felt pain in his midback. He took analgesics and did not get evaluated for this problem. A year later he was found to have two vertebral fractures and a DXA demonstrating a T score of −3. He was instructed to take calcium, vitamin D, and started on teriparatide therapy. Within two months, his back pain improved. Within a year, a repeat DXA demonstrated an improved T score of −2.6.

## Future Therapy

RANK ligand (RANKL) is a chemical that causes cells to become osteoclasts. Blocking RANKL results in fewer osteoclasts and less leeching away of bone calcium. Denosumab is a monoclonal antibody that blocks the RANKL receptor. The result is less bone resorption and an increase in bone density in the hip, spine, and forearm to a similar degree as alendronate. The drug is given as an injection approximately every six months.

## REGAINING HEIGHT

Patients who develop acute fractures of vertebral bodies may lose height. If the fractures are adequately severe or numerous, you can develop a significant curvature in the spine. In addition, these fractures are acutely painful such that every breath can hurt.

Medical therapy for this problem is the use of analgesics, intranasal calcitonin, and initiation of drug therapy for osteoporosis. You may find this therapy perfectly adequate to relieve your pain. However, a concern may remain that a curvature exists or that your back pain has not been controlled.

Invasive procedures, in the form of vertebroplasty for old fractures, and kyphoplasty, for acute fractures, are available for persistent pain and deformity. Patients with healed osteoporotic fractures after six to eight weeks of healing may have persistent spine pain. Vertebroplasty is a procedure where bone cement is forced with high pressure into the collapsed vertebral body for structural support. The added cement is placed to stabilize the area with the expectation of decreased spine pain. The potential harm of the procedure is that the need for high pressure may cause a fracture of the bone with the spread of bone cement into the spinal canal. A spine surgery is needed to remove the cement if this fracture occurs.

Kyphoplasty is performed in a vertebral body up to eight weeks from the time of fracture. The procedure can be done before the fracture has fully healed. An inflatable balloon is passed into the flattened vertebral body and is inflated to restore height. The expanded space is filled with bone cement under low pressure, minimizing the risk of additional fracture by the cement. Studies have demonstrated the benefit of kyphoplasty for the relief of acute fracture pain compared to medical therapy alone. However, you need to have drug therapy started for osteoporosis if you require a kyphoplasty. By definition, a vertebral fracture means you have osteoporosis. Concerns remain that if you are not treated for osteoporosis, you may be at risk of additional vertebral fractures because of the presence of spine cement.

## PREVENTING FALLS

The best treatment for osteoporosis remains prevention. Falls are a big concern, particularly in the elderly. Our houses are filled with potential hazards in almost every room.

Remember to remove throw rugs that slip. Place railings on tubs, toilet areas, and stairways. Install nonslip surfaces on showers and tubs. Have good lighting in areas that include stairs. Clear clutter from walkways. As far as osteoporosis is concerned, an ounce of prevention is worth a pound of cure.

---

### DR. B'S PRESCRIPTION SUMMARY

- Osteoporosis is a common medical problem associated with increased disability and mortality.
- Risk factors for osteoporosis include increased age, family history, being female, and smoking.
- A DXA test is the easiest means to determine bone mineral density (BMD). A T score of -2.5 is the BMD associated with osteoporosis.
- BMD can be maintained with weight-bearing exercise and taking calcium and vitamin D supplements.
- Drug therapy in the form of **SERMs**, calcitonin, bisphosphonates, or parathyroid hormones can improve BMD and decrease risk of fracture.
- Kyphoplasty is a surgical therapy to restore height and decrease pain with spinal fractures of less than eight weeks in duration.
- Preventing falls by removing obstacles, improving lighting, and installing hand rails is important in preventing fractures.

---

# Chapter 8

# Back Pain in Kids

## *Is It Just Growing Pains or Is It More Serious?*

BACK PAIN DOES AFFECT children, but a little less frequently than adults. In young children under ten about 30 percent have an episode of back pain, while about 50 percent of adolescents from fifteen on have had the complaint. Most episodes of back pain resolve spontaneously in children over a time period measured in weeks. If back pain persists in a child more than four to six weeks, a doctor should evaluate the child. Most back pain in children is mechanical, just like it is in adults. Spondylolysis and spondylolisthesis are fractures of part of the vertebral body and start during teenage years, particularly in divers and gymnasts. Disc herniations are extremely rare. Systemic illnesses, such as infections, tumors, and sickle cell disease, do occur in children but are unusual. The red flags for more serious illnesses are the same for adults and children. Psychological problems related to peer pressure and emotional difficulties may play as important a role as mechanical disorders as a source of back pain in a significant proportion of children.

### GROWING PAINS

Exactly what are growing pains and are they benign or a sign of serious illness? The answer is that growing pains are crampy sensations in the lower extremities in the thigh, shin, or calf. Growing pains do not usually affect the back. They occur at night and often interrupt sleep. They resolve by the morning or can respond to massage or aspirin-like drugs. Physical activity is normal during the day. Almost 20 percent of school-aged children may have growing pains. In the vast majority of children, these nighttime episodes disappear.

## NONSPECIFIC LOW BACK PAIN

The vast majority of children and adolescents with an episode of back pain have a benign condition that will resolve spontaneously. In most circumstances, the source of the pain cannot be identified. The soft tissues around the spine are likely candidates. No laboratory test or X ray technique exists to identify these locations. Episodes of back pain may occur more than once. Recurrent events are not uncommon. These episodes resolve without damage to the spine. They are not associated with back problems as adults.

### Frustrated Teenager

Jane is a fourteen-year-old field hockey player with a four-month history of back pain. She was frustrated by the fact that she wanted to play her sport but had pain any time she started to bend backward. She had seen her pediatrician who had ordered X rays that were normal. She had tried a small amount of ibuprofen without success. She had not done any exercises for fear of making her back worse. Her examination showed a calm, but concerned female who had increased pain and muscle tension with any backward motion of the spine. She had mild limitation of motion of her spine. She was told that she would get better but it would take some time. She was given a longer-acting NSAID and a muscle relaxant in the evening. She was sent to physical therapy for strengthening exercises for the core muscles of the abdomen and back. She was pleased to see an improvement in her symptoms within four weeks. She was particularly happy when she returned to playing her sport the next season knowing the importance of her exercises to protect her back.

Psychological problems have become recognized as a major source of back pain in adolescents. Depression and other emotional distress may be manifested as low back pain. Stress from peer pressure may also be a causative factor. Back pain may also be associated with headaches or abdominal complaints. These young adults require emotional support to discuss their concerns.

## KIDS' RED FLAGS

Children who have fever, a limp, or weight loss do not have "usual" growing pains. These children are more likely to have a serious illness and should be evaluated. Back pain in children four years or younger is associated with anatomic abnormalities or systemic illness more commonly than in adolescents. Discitis is an inflammation of an intervertebral disc that is caused by bacteria. Children between the ages of one to four seem to be at particular risk. Antibiotics are the therapy for this disorder. Tumors of the spine or nervous system also appear in young children more commonly. For example, about 6 percent of children with leukemia have back pain as a complaint.

Inflammatory arthritis of the spine causes persistent low back pain. Teenage years are when these disorders appear. Increasing stiffness becomes a common complaint. These individuals may have other joints involved like knees or hips. They may also have complaints of fever, weight loss, or change of bowel habits. Evaluation by a rheumatologist can identify the presence of spondyloarthropathy. A number of therapies, including biologics, are available to treat this arthritis effectively.

## ADOLESCENT SCOLIOSIS

Scoliosis is an abnormal lateral curvature of the spine that may also have a rotational component. Adolescent idiopathic scoliosis accounts for upward of 85 percent of all individuals with this problem. The addition of idiopathic to the name of the disorder signifies that no specific reason is known to cause the curvature. Adolescent idiopathic scoliosis starts after age ten. Identification of the problem prior to periods of rapid skeletal growth is important to minimize the development of significant deformity.

Many adolescents with scoliosis are pain-free and are identified in screening clinics at school. Children who complain of pain are more likely to have a nonidiopathic form of the structural abnormality. Therefore, the presence of scoliosis and pain is worthy of an evaluation to rule out the presence of an underlying pathologic condition such as malformations of the spinal cord.

Another concern is early-onset scoliosis in children up to nine years of age. Congenital and neuromuscular problems affect these younger children. Congenital abnormalities occur when babies are born with spines that do not develop with the appropriate number or shape of vertebra. Neuromuscular problems result in loss of muscle control such as those associated with cerebral palsy or muscular dystrophy. These are the curves with the greatest risk of progression.

Figure 8.1.    Cobb's angle is
65 degrees in this example.

Cobb's angle is a measurement of the curvature of the spine from upright. (See fig. 8.1.) Spines with a Cobb's angle of 10 degrees or greater are considered scoliotic. Only about 3 percent of adolescents have a Cobb's angle greater than 10. Only a small proportion of individuals with adolescent scoliosis (0.3 percent) actually require treatment.

Individuals with angles of 20 degrees benefit from an evaluation by a specialist. Curves may stabilize at any point but do tend to progress once they are associated with a Cobb's angle of 40 or more. These individuals may progress 1 degree per year. The greatest health concern is difficulty breathing if movement of the chest is limited by the spinal curve.

### Straightening the Curve

Great controversy exists over the correct therapy for adolescent idiopathic scoliosis. Studies observing adolescent scoliosis patients for fifty years with no therapy demonstrate a mild increase in back pain but no increase in mortality.

Bracing does not correct scoliosis but may prevent progression. Therefore, bracing is indicated for children who are young enough to have a growth spurt. Scoliosis can progress a degree a month during growth spurts. The TLSO (thoraco-lumbar-sacral orthosis) brace is worn under the arms under clothing. The general recommendation is for twenty-three hours per day of use. In most studies the brace is worn 65 percent of the recommended time. The brace is worn until the end of growth about twenty-four months after the start of menstrual periods.

Surgical therapy for idiopathic scoliosis is undertaken to prevent the progression of spine deformity that will result in mechanical disability. Surgical correction is considered for individuals with Cobb's angles between 40 to 50 degrees. In the past Harrington rods that spanned a number of thoracic and lumbar vertebrae were used. Current surgical techniques have preferred segmental corrections with shorter rods connecting fewer vertebrae. This technique offers a better opportunity for positioning the spine. The goal of scoliosis surgery is completing a bony fusion of the spine. The bone used for the fusion may come from your own pelvis, or from a cadaver donor. The success of surgeries from the standpoint of fusion is about 95 percent. Complications of scoliosis surgery include nerve injury, infection, implant failure, and fusion failure. Surgically treated scoliosis patients have a halt in the progression of spinal curvature but tend to have more back pain than nonsurgically treated individuals when examined twenty years or more after their procedures.

## ADOLESCENT DOWAGER'S HUMP—SCHEUERMANN'S DISEASE

Girls between the age of thirteen and seventeen who develop a round shoulder posture with a dowager's hump (fig. 2.2) have Scheuermann's disease. This condition is caused either by weakening of the front of the vertebral body causing a wedge deformity or overgrowth of the posterior wall of the vertebrae. In either circumstance, the vertebral body, instead of looking like a rectangle, takes on the shape of a slice of pizza. Up to three or more neighboring vertebral bodies are affected causing the round-shouldered appearance. The anterior wedging is thought to occur because the gel from the neighboring intervertebral disc invades the vertebral body. The replacement of bone with disc gel weakens the bone allowing for fracture of bone. The increase in the chest curve is reflected in an increased curve in the lumbar spine. Patients with Scheuermann's disease have pain in the thoracic and lumbar spine. Usually, the treatment is anti-inflammatory therapy and the use of a brace to prevent an increase in forward movement of the spine. Most teenagers become adults without significant disability related to this condition. Surgery to correct the forward bend of the spine is limited to individuals who are in a position looking at the floor.

## ADOLESCENT SPONDYLOLISTHESIS

Cartilage plates allow for the growth of bone while we are young, and one such plate exists in the extension of the vertebrae between the joints. As we mature, our bones become solid and these cartilage plates close. Spondylolysis and spondylolisthesis occur because of a crack in this back section of a vertebra. This abnormality occurs in about 6 percent of the population but goes undetected because the lesion may develop without pain.

If physical activities during childhood, such as gymnastics, which involves bending backward, cause enough strain on this cartilage plate, the plate will not close. This is a spondylolysis. If enough strain is placed on the cartilage plate, then the front end of the vertebra, which is no longer attached to the back part of the vertebra, may move forward. This instability is a spondylolisthesis, commonly known as a slipped vertebra (see fig. 5.2). This instability occurs most frequently at the L5 interspace. Because these spinal abnormalities occur during active growth in childhood, they are called developmental spondylolisthesis. For some, this instability remains painless throughout life. Even physically active individuals, such as football players, may remain free of pain. You may be unaware of the presence of a spondylolisthesis, but it may be identified by chance when an X ray is taken of the abdomen or spine for another reason.

Therapy of developmental spondylolysis depends on the time of its discovery. Some young individuals with new-onset back pain in the setting of sports activities have undergone bone scan or MRI scans to identify the status of the fracture. Acute fractures can heal when the two ends of the fracture are placed together. These individuals will benefit from a hard brace worn continuously for three months. Repeat scans in these individuals can document fusion of the fractures. Other individuals are identified when the ends of the bone near the fracture have already healed. For these individuals the ends of the fracture will not fuse and result in a pseudoarthrosis. These individuals may return to sports activities once their pain is relieved. Most individuals are not at risk for greater slippage of the vertebral bodies at the fractured level. In those adults where pain persists despite drug therapy and strengthening exercises, surgical fusion is successful in the majority to allow a return to activities of daily living without back pain.

### Backpacks and Back Pain

A current problem affecting children of all ages is what they are wearing on their backs. More and more kids of school age are having back problems because of excessively heavy backpacks and book bags. These heavy bags strain the muscles of the back and cause fatigue that aches. You can see some kids waiting at the bus stop bent over from the weight on their backs.

Book bags should not weigh more than 15 to 20 percent of the child's weight. If they are too heavy, lighten them up. The bag should have adjustable straps. The bag should be worn over both shoulders. The shoulders should carry most of the weight. Bags hanging too high or too low on the back place strain across the lumbar spine, increasing low back pain. The good aspect of wearing the right weight backpack is that it is exercise. Carrying weights is one of the ways children are able to get exercise just going to school. With an epidemic of obesity and too many hours of video games, using up calories carrying the correct weight can be a good thing even though the time each day is usually short.

---

### DR. B'S PRESCRIPTION SUMMARY

- Low back pain is a common complaint of children.
- Nonspecific low back pain is the most common category.
- Psychological factors (peer stress) may play a significant role as a source of the problem.
- Red flags are similar in adults and children particularly in those four years and younger.
- The vast majority of episodes resolve without the need for an evaluation by a physician.
- Most curves of the spine do not require surgery. Only those that compromise breathing require correction.
- Backpacks have their good and bad aspects. Weight in packs can be a good source of exercise. Do not make the packs so heavy as to cause back strain.

---

# Chapter 9

# How and When to Use
# Medications Effectively for Pain

FOR THE MAJORITY OF PEOPLE with back pain from mechanical disorders, a single drug is adequate to decrease pain. But the more inflammatory the problem, the greater the need for a combination of drug categories. Trial and error determine the best combination, and both patients and physicians can tire of this process, which unfortunately may lead to inadequate therapy. With some patients, I have tried ten different medications before finding the one that is effective and tolerated. I persisted because a drug regimen is so important in the prescription for low back pain. No single drug therapy is effective for all illnesses that cause spinal disease and pain. NSAIDs and analgesics have been proven effective for acute low back pain, but many back pain sufferers are resistant to using these medications even when the drugs make them feel better.

When I prescribed physical therapy and an NSAID to Chet, a forty-year-old carpenter, he refused the medication because he didn't want it to hide the pain and therefore lead to greater muscle damage. I explained to Chet that without relieving pain he would not be able to get the maximum benefit from his exercises. In his case, the prescription for his low back pain would be incomplete if he didn't agree to use the medications. If he performed his exercises with gradually increasing intensity and duration, the likelihood of causing extra muscle damage was small. Chet eventually relented and realized the NSAID allowed him to carry out his exercise program, and over the next month, his back pain disappeared. At that point he was able to stop taking the drug. As long as he continues his exercises, he can do his work. Chet's case is an example of the importance of looking at a back treatment prescription as an integrated whole, not just a group of options.

Many people are like Chet. They assume it's essential to feel pain in order to gauge improvement. This is simply not true. Drugs often effectively control pain while the underlying problem is improving. However, the medications do not always cure the underlying problem and once the medication is discontinued the pain may recur. Remember, too, that people with medical conditions that produce pain, such as arthritis, have used NSAIDs for decades without ill effects.

Even though NSAIDs and analgesics are not habit-forming opioids, people may believe they are "addicted" to these medicines and dislike this sense of dependency. Mixed messages about drugs are all around us. On one hand, we hear the messages about illegal drugs and we are urged to work toward a "drug-free" society. On the other hand, we greatly value drugs with legitimate medical uses. How many lives would have been lost if antibiotics had not been developed? Sometimes patients confuse apples and oranges, and their concern about drugs in general adds to the stress associated with pain.

This fear of dependency is one reason people stop taking their pain medications too soon. Twenty-eight-year-old Lowell is a good example. He was in constant pain from a muscle strain caused by a skiing accident. This was aggravated when he twisted his spine, a motion his work required. In addition, not being able to ski for the two years since his accident both frustrated and depressed him. Exercises had not improved his condition.

Lowell was afraid of becoming dependent on a drug in order to feel well, and he also was concerned about stomach irritation. I started him on a medication from one of the newer classes of drugs, the COX-2 inhibitors, and when it was clear that Lowell tolerated the drug, I increased his daily dose. In a short time his back pain resolved, along with full movement of his spine, and his blood tests were normal and showed no toxicity from his drug.

Two months later Lowell planned his first ski trip since his injury. However, his continued concern about his "drug dependency" led him to stop the medicine for a few days. Predictably, his pain returned. I reassured Lowell that even after taking the drug for four months, he was not "addicted" to his medicine. He proved that to himself because he had stopped the medicine without any difficulty other than a return of his back pain. Furthermore, I could not tell him exactly how long he would need to take this medicine before his back pain resolved. I also emphasized that his ability to go on the ski trip was due to the effectiveness of the medication. After all, maximizing function is the primary goal of therapy. Taking a medication is the price we pay for function—and I believe it is a reasonable cost. Lowell took his medicine during his trip and was able to enjoy skiing again.

## NSAIDs AND COX-2 INHIBITORS

NSAIDs are nonsteroidal anti-inflammatory drugs, and they comprise the most frequently prescribed class of medicines. They are indicated for a variety of musculoskeletal diseases that affect the spine, including muscle injuries, herniated discs, osteoarthritis, and AS. NSAIDs reduce fever, pain, swelling, and clotting. These drugs are analgesic (painkillers) when taken in single doses. In larger doses over a longer period of time, they are also anti-inflammatory. Side effects include irritation to the stomach lining and—in very rare cases—stomach pain, holes in the intestinal wall, bowel blockage, and kidney failure.

Toxic side effects can be monitored with blood tests for liver and kidney function. The frequency of blood tests depends on your underlying health status. For example, young, healthy adults taking NSAIDs on a daily basis need blood tests once a year; older people with multiple medical problems may require monthly blood tests. While these NSAID-associated toxic effects are real, they are also manageable.

COX-2 inhibitors have similar efficacy to NSAIDs but have the potential to decrease gastrointestinal irritation. Here's why: the production of hormone-like substances called prostaglandins (PGs) can be inhibited by an enzyme called **cyclooxygenase** (COX). Originally, a single COX enzyme was thought to regulate the production of PGs for the purpose of maintaining stomach lining and generating an inflammatory response. The NSAIDs decrease COX-1 activity, thus increasing the risk for stomach ulcers, leg swelling, and the bleeding associated with decreased platelet function. The degree to which normal functions are inhibited varies and is an individual response.

When a second COX enzyme was discovered, this advanced our understanding of the way NSAIDs work. COX-1 is present all the time and produces PGs that maintain organ function, including the stomach lining, blood pressure, and the airways in the lungs, and it helps maintain the correct balance of fluid in the body. COX-2 is an enzyme produced at sites of inflammation. The prostaglandins produced by COX-2 are associated with heat and swelling, and redness and pain in affected areas. When we inhibit COX-2 we can control inflammation and pain to about the same degree as occurred with the older NSAIDs, but with less toxicity. So the new COX-2 inhibitors are "safer aspirin," not "super aspirin."

COX-2 inhibitors have been proven to be safer in regard to gastrointestinal toxicity, halving the risk for significant bleeding. COX-2 agents have kidney toxicities similar to the aspirin-like drugs. Similar to older NSAIDs, COX-2 inhibitors can diminish renal function, causing swelling in the feet and increasing blood pressure. Questions remain regarding effects of COX-2 on the heart. Platelets cause clotting, which can result in heart attack. COX-2 inhibitors have no effect on platelet function; therefore, COX-2 inhibitors do not prevent heart attacks. But that does not mean they promote heart attacks. You should speak to your doctor about your health status and decide which combination of drugs is best for your condition.

### Finding the Right NSAID for Your Pain

NSAIDs and COX-2 inhibitors currently available for the treatment of spinal disorders are listed in appendix B. The choice and dosage of NSAIDs depend on factors related to your medical condition. Acute mechanical conditions (muscle strain) occurring in young people require NSAIDs with rapid onset of action and pain-relieving properties, such as ibuprofen, naproxen, ketoprofen, and diclofenac potassium. For these acute mechanical disorders, treatment with NSAIDs generally lasts two to four weeks. Concerns about toxicity are less significant if, for example, you are young with a muscle strain that will improve in a short period and you do not have any other medical problems.

NSAIDs available over the counter (OTC) include ibuprofen (Advil, Motrin IB, Nuprin), naproxen (Aleve), and ketoprofen (Orudis KT). These same drugs are available in prescription strength: Motrin, Naprelan, and Orudis, respectively. If the OTC products are taken in high doses, they will have the same benefits and toxicities as their prescription counterparts. These over-the-counter medications have a lower, but continued, risk of toxicity. Since most adults routinely take these products for minor pain, the best advice I can give you is to follow the instructions on the pill container, but if your symptoms do not subside, see your doctor. Do not take more without your doctor's advice.

Aspirin, a powerful NSAID, improves low back pain and is effective but potentially toxic. The same properties that make aspirin effective for preventing heart attacks and strokes also increase the risk for bleeding. In addition to stomach ulcers, aspirin can cause ringing in the ears, reversible deafness, and death if taken in a high dosage. Never exceed the recommended dose without advice from your doctor.

Use a COX-2 inhibitor if you have a history of stomach ulcers. If you are taking either an NSAID or COX-2 inhibitor on a daily basis, you should have your weight and blood pressure measured regularly. Some NSAIDs can increase fluid retention and blood pressure, and blood tests also are indicated to monitor for toxicities affecting blood counts and kidney and liver function.

### Understanding Timing and Dosage

Dosages of NSAIDs and COX-2 inhibitors vary based on the length of time they stay in your body. This is known as the drug's half-life. For example, NSAIDs that are eliminated from the body more slowly require fewer pills per day for a sustained anti-inflammatory effect. NSAIDs and COX-2 inhibitors with long half-lives include piroxicam, oxaprozin, celecoxib, and meloxicam. Some NSAIDs are eliminated rapidly but can be given once or twice a day in sustained release formulations. Examples include naproxen, ketoprofen, etodolac, indomethacin, and diclofenac.

If a medication helps for a portion of the day but then loses effect, an additional dose at the end of a day may be appropriate. If a drug is somewhat toxic, it may be easier on you if you limit your intake of alcohol and coffee. Smoking can also exacerbate drug toxicities. If NSAIDs are not effective, and if you have a history of stomach ulcers or if you take corticosteroids, you are an appropriate candidate for COX-2 inhibitors.

NSAIDs and COX-2 inhibitors come in different sizes and forms, including tablets, capsules, and liquids. The pills may be small or large. All these factors may play a role in deciding which drug is best for you. For example, celecoxib comes in 100 mg and 200 mg tablets. The dosage for an older person with osteoarthritis might be 200 mg, while someone with severe pain might be taking 800 mg a day. Celecoxib has greatest activity in the body over an eleven-hour period and is usually prescribed twice a day. However, for many people, a 200 mg tablet once a day is adequate to control the symptoms of arthritis.

NSAIDs should be taken with food to decrease stomach toxicities, but COX-2 inhibitors can be taken on an empty stomach. You should review the doses of all your medications, and how you take them, with your physician.

The future is uncertain regarding more effective and safer COX-2 inhibitors. These medicines should offer more anti-inflammatory effects with less toxicity than currently available COX-2 inhibitors. One COX-2 inhibitor, etoricoxib, is available in other parts of the world, but has not been released by the Food and Drug Administration for distribution in the United States. This drug continues to be evaluated to determine its place as an addition to therapies currently available.

Concerns remain in the determination of the risk-benefit balance for NSAIDs and COX-2 inhibitors. NSAIDs and COX-2 inhibitors offer anti-inflammatory and pain-relieving therapy. This is a difficult combination of benefits to find in other categories of drugs or natural supplements. At the same time, these agents are associated with infrequent but real risks that can cause harm. Attempts have been made to correlate the risk of taking an NSAID with other life events, like riding a motorcycle. I find using these analogies with my patients does not work. Most patients just want to know if it is worth the risk. They value the doctor's opinion, but remain skeptical and cautious.

When I first started caring for patients in the 1970s, my patients asked for the medicine that worked. In 2010, my patients ask for the medicine that is safe. Over this period of decades, the pendulum has swung widely from a concern with efficacy to an almost exclusive concern with safety. The pendulum should be in the middle. I tell my patients that if a drug is not effective, they do not need to worry about whether it is safe because they will not be taking it. Safety needs to be maximized once the efficacy of the drug is established. The toxicities of the NSAIDs and COX-2 inhibitors are known. For example, heart attacks do not occur immediately after starting one of these medicines.

The development of hypertension is the most likely cause of cardiovascular events associated with this class of drug. Blood pressure can be monitored to limit the exposure to any increase related to drugs. You may be asked to change your diet, to limit salt intake, for example. Or lose weight to lower blood pressure. By making thoughtful choices, you may have the benefit of using these medicines to decrease your pain while limiting your risks. Over time, additional research will need to be conducted to define their benefits and guide us as we determine their future role in pain management.

## Smear It On

What if you could apply your medicine to the place that hurts? You could have the benefit of pain relief without the general body exposure of using the same medicine by mouth.

A number of topical forms of NSAID therapy are now available that can be placed on a painful low back. The drugs are available as a gel, solution, or patch. Diclofenac is the NSAID that is most frequently utilized as a topical medicine. As a gel or lotion, applications may be needed four times a day to get adequate relief. NSAID patches are applied every twelve hours for benefit. Theoretically, the medicine in the gel and patches sinks into a painful, inflamed area just below the skin. How a topical medicine helps tissues that are inches below the surface is not clear. In many circumstances it seems to work without causing side effects.

Isabel is an eighty-year-old woman with intermittent low back pain. Her back pain is increased when she stands for long periods of time. She has used acetaminophen with modest benefit. She has a history of stomach ulcers and is concerned about the use of aspirin-like drugs by mouth that could cause a return of her ulcers. She was informed about the availability of diclofenac gel that she could apply over the painful area as needed. She returned a month later with a smile on her face. She was skeptical, but the gel worked. She would put the gel on and let it dry for eight minutes about three times a day. She found that the gel helped her pain and did not cause any gastrointestinal (GI) distress. She would use the gel when she needed it.

Another form of topical therapy is topical lidocaine. Lidocaine is an anesthetic when injected. The same medicine can calm skipped heart beats when given intravenously. When applied to the skin, the Lidoderm (lidocaine) patch will release the anesthetic for twelve hours as it attaches to pain receptors that are generated on the endings of sensory nerves. Most commonly, lidocaine patches are applied to the skin during a shingles attack. Shingles or herpes zoster is the chicken pox virus that reemerges as an adult. If you have back pain independent of shingles, the pain fibers over the surface of the back have increased pain receptors. Applying a Lidoderm patch every day has the potential to offer pain relief without oral medicines. Up to three patches may be used at one time.

Remember, NSAIDs can be effective in a number of different forms. Although there are risks, the benefits of this class of drug are worth it in most individuals. Learn about the drugs for your situation. You may find that they are the missing component of therapy that offers significant relief of pain.

## MUSCLE RELAXANTS

The Agency for Healthcare Research and Quality (AHRQ) has reviewed studies of muscle relaxants and concluded that they are probably as helpful as NSAIDs for low back pain, but they cause drowsiness in 30 percent of those taking them and are prescribed infrequently. However, studies have shown that muscle relaxants, particularly cyclobenzaprine, can have a beneficial effect without causing drowsiness in the vast majority of individuals who benefit from the drug.

I have found that muscle relaxants are particularly helpful for muscle strain and its associated spasm. A study from a health maintenance organization in the state of Washington reported that an NSAID and a muscle relaxant were the most effective combination of medications for people with acute low back pain. Muscle relaxants can also be effective for chronic low back pain when you have limited motion because of muscle tightness.

The combination of NSAIDs and muscle relaxants is effective for reversing the "pain-spasm cycle," characterized by muscle pain that causes increasing muscle spasm, and thus, more pain and more spasm. An analgesic and muscle relaxant allows treatment of both components of the cycle. Treating just one component of the cycle may not correct the problem because either the pain or the spasm persists. A complete prescription requires both classes of drugs if you have muscle spasm.

We still do not know exactly how muscle relaxants work, but we do know they do not work directly on the muscles in the arms and legs. Their effect is on the central nervous system, which controls the tension in muscles. Thus, they work to calm tension in the damaged muscle.

Like NSAIDs, beneficial response to muscle relaxants varies with the individual and so trial and error is sometimes necessary. I usually start patients on the lowest dose, taken two hours before sleep. Since the action of most muscle relaxants is delayed, taking them in the evening before sleep eliminates problems created by drowsiness. Muscle relaxants currently available are listed in appendix B.

## Incapacitated Mother

Lucy's back pain had a detrimental effect on her work as a computer programmer but also made it difficult to take care of her twelve-year-old child. She had so much difficulty walking that her twelve-year-old daughter was helping her put on her clothes and doing all the household chores. Lucy was becoming increasingly concerned about the burden her daughter was carrying. She was supposed to be practicing the violin, not taking care of her mother.

Examination revealed a severe degree of muscle spasm in the right buttock and lower back muscles. Although she had received NSAIDs in the past, she had never been given a muscle relaxant. I prescribed cyclobenzaprine (Flexeril), three times a day, along with her naproxen. Within two weeks, her back pain had decreased, and although she was still stiff, she was able to take over more of the household chores. Lucy also started a stretching exercise program, and within another month she returned to work. Drug doses decreased over the next year, and she eventually used exercises exclusively as the means to control her pain and was able to sit comfortably at her daughter's violin recital.

A wide range of muscle relaxants is available. These drugs are used while increased muscle spasm and decreased range of motion are present and quickly withdrawn once muscle spasm is resolved. Some of the medications include cyclobenzaprine (Flexeril), orphenadrine (Norflex), chlorzoxazone (Parafon Forte), and metaxalone (Skelaxin). These medications may cause drowsiness. Flexeril is available in a 5 mg tablet. The smaller tablet works well to decrease spasm and has less toxicity than the 10 mg form of the drug.

A long-acting form of cyclobenzaprine can be taken once a day. Amrix is available in 15 and 30 mg capsules. The capsule contains many individual pellets of the medicine that dissolve over a specific time period. The medicine is to be taken at about 6 to 7 p.m. The maximum concentration is reached at about midnight. The concentration gradually decreases as individuals awaken in the morning. A lower level of medicine is maintained during the day. This limits the potential for increased sleepiness during the day.

I do not use the antianxiety drug diazepam (Valium) because, unlike other muscle relaxants, it has a tendency to cause depression when used for a long time. I also use carisoprodol (Soma) less often than other muscle relaxants. It has properties of a sedative. Some patients require increasing doses for a beneficial effect. Discontinuing cariso-prodol can be difficult when these increased doses have been utilized.

## OPIOID AND NONOPIOID ANALGESICS

If you are unable to tolerate NSAIDs, you may benefit from analgesics. The pure analgesics reduce pain but have no effect on a disease's inflammatory component and, therefore, are not preferred therapy in many circumstances. Pain-relieving medications—analgesics—are divided into nonopioid and opioid groups.

### Nonopioid Analgesics

Acetaminophen (Tylenol) is a pure analgesic without any anti-inflammatory effects. It works by decreasing PG production in the central nervous system but has no effect on the production of PG in the rest of the body. Acetaminophen is a less-effective analgesic than aspirin, but it has none of the toxic side effects such as stomach ulcers or breathing difficulties associated with the NSAIDs. If you have aspirin sensitivity, acetaminophen should be the first pain therapy you take. It should also be considered if you are older and have osteoarthritis of the spine. It can be used in combination with NSAIDs or opioid drugs.

Check with your physician to determine the maximum dose of acetaminophen that is appropriate for your clinical condition. Be especially cautious if you drink alcohol on a daily basis and take acetaminophen, because both drugs can affect liver function. If you drink alcohol regularly, you must speak with your doctor before you use acetaminophen or other pain relievers. Taking more than the recommended dose may cause severe liver damage.

Acetaminophen is available in a variety of doses (325 mg, 500 mg, 650 mg) and forms (tablets, capsules, liquid). Acetaminophen extended-release is special in that the effect of the medicine is prolonged. Where the effect of regular acetaminophen is about four hours, the extended-release form is dissolved more slowly and has a six- to eight-hour effect. Taken three times a day, this drug is able to offer pain relief around the clock.

Tramadol (Ultram) is another nonopioid, pure analgesic that is as effective as aspirin and ibuprofen. Its action is mediated through activation of opioid and serotonin receptors in the central nervous system. Like acetaminophen, tramadol has no cross-reaction with NSAIDs, and if you are sensitive to aspirin you can take tramadol without concern about difficulty breathing. This drug also has no effect on the stomach lining, although tramadol may cause nausea and dizziness. Do not take tramadol if you have a history of seizures, because it lowers the seizure threshold, thereby increasing the risk of seizure occurrence.

Tramadol comes as a 50 mg tablet that can be broken into 25 mg halves. You should start the drug at 25 mg to decrease the risk of nausea. You can increase the dose as tolerated after consultation with your physician. Most people benefit at less than the maximum dose. Like acetaminophen, tramadol is synergistic and can be used with NSAIDs for additional pain relief. The drug may be given up to four times a day.

Long-acting forms of tramadol are available. The convenience of these medicines is that they can be given once a day with efficacy extending twenty-four hours. This form of tramadol is supplied in 100, 200, and 300 mg tablets. Once you have tried tramadol to know that it is effective and tolerable you can have the convenience of taking the medicine once a day. Once-a-day dosing improves compliance with the drug.

Ultracet is a combination of 37.5 mg tramadol and 325 mg acetaminophen that lasts longer and has greater pain-relieving properties than the individual drug components.

New agents are available that have dual action, like tramadol, but have greater pain relieving properties. Tapentadol (Nucynta) is available in 50, 75, and 100 mg tablets. This agent is listed as a Schedule II drug, similar to opioid therapies. A risk of possible dependence needs to be considered if the drug is prescribed other than for short-term use. Tapentadol may have an advantage over other Schedule II drugs with a lower risk of nausea and constipation.

### Opioid Analgesics

Opioid medicines are **narcotics.** You do not need opioid analgesics such as codeine, hydrocodone, meperidine, morphine, or fentanyl to treat the usual episode of acute low back pain. However, if you have severe sciatica related to a herniated disc, opioid analgesics, used along with NSAIDs and muscle relaxants, are part of your complete prescription to ease pain. The risk of developing dependency is the major toxicity of opioids, so they are stopped as soon as possible. Opioid drugs work by attaching to the receptors in the pain-reducing pathway in the central nervous system.

Opioid analgesics are of limited use for treating chronic low back pain. In the past, opioids needed to be given every few hours because their analgesic effects wore off quickly. Opioid drugs with prolonged action have been developed, including OxyContin, Kadian, MS Contin, and Duragesic. These drugs can be dosed orally twice a day or in patch form once every three days. The long duration of the patch allows for sustained pain relief with decreased toxicities.

These opioid analgesics improve physical function of chronic pain patients with failed back surgery (see chapter 12) and those with direct nerve damage associated with persistent sciatica. The dose of drug is increased until pain is controlled. Increasing the dose beyond this level of pain control does not increase the efficacy of the drug, but it does increase the risk of toxicity. In addition to dependency, opioids cause constipation and sleepiness.

Fortunately, relatively few people require chronic opioid therapy, but for those individuals, these drugs are essential for a functional quality of life. Both you and your physician should be comfortable with the choice before committing to chronic, long-acting opioid therapy. You and your physician must review the benefits and detriments of these drugs before you start taking them. While opioids do not always make people "high," some of these drugs depress mood, and they can cause headaches, disorientation, and constipation. You may be asked to sign an opioid therapy contract that describes the conditions under which the drug will be prescribed and your responsibilities as a patient to take the opioid in an appropriate manner.

Debates are ongoing concerning the benefits and risks of sustained opioid therapy. Studies have reported that prolonged opioid therapy may result in alterations in the nervous system pathways that process pain signals. Opioids may dull their own benefits on the nerve cells that inhibit pain. Theses modifications may result in decreasing pain relief. When this modification occurs is not known. The possibility of a negative response needs to be considered as chronic opioid therapy is initiated.

Codeine is a frequently prescribed opioid. However, it is relatively weak and causes gastrointestinal distress with nausea. Other opioids, such as oxycodone or hydrocodone, in varying combinations with aspirin or acetaminophen, are useful to decrease pain in the appropriate individuals. The goal is to decrease the use of these medications as soon as pain is decreased. A listing of opioids is included in appendix B.

# CORTICOSTEROIDS

Glucocorticoids, such as prednisone, are not related to androgenic steroids that athletes take to build muscles, and they are not toxic. Your body actually makes the equivalent of 7.5 mg of prednisone every day. The difference is that the body-made corticosteroids are released all day long whereas the pharmaceutical prednisone is absorbed all at one time.

Some people fear steroid medication because they have heard that common side effects are increased appetite and weight gain, but this does not happen to everyone. I tell my patients there are no calories in the pills. Eating a healthy diet can improve the chances of maintaining your weight without gaining. Other side effects include high blood pressure, cataracts, diabetes, and osteoporosis, but these problems come with long-term use. Always discuss side effects with your physician, because once recognized, they can be treated.

Oral corticosteroids are reserved for people with severe pain or muscle weakness that has not improved with NSAIDs alone. The decision to use corticosteroids should be made after your entire medical condition is reviewed. I prefer to order low doses of prednisone for an extended period of time. Other physicians prefer a larger dose of corticosteroids, which is then tapered over a seven-day course. Low doses for a short period of time reduce potential toxic side effects. Once improvement is achieved, the steroids are tapered. If no improvement occurs at four weeks, the steroids are quickly discontinued.

In rare circumstances, a low dose of prednisone may be used to treat spinal stenosis. Patients who are resistant to epidural injections (see following discussion), have had maximum NSAID therapy, and have refused decompression surgery generally remain incapacitated, even unable to walk short distances. In these very specialized circumstances, low-dose prednisone may be helpful.

Response to the drug needs to be constantly monitored. If signs of improvement disappear, the medicine should be discontinued.

### Stay-at-Home Octogenarian

Evelyn is an eighty-two-year-old woman with a number of medical problems including diabetes and associated moderate kidney failure, leg swelling, and spinal stenosis that limits her walking. She was concerned because she had difficulty getting around her house. She was afraid that unless something was done, she was going to have to leave her home. She had tried acetaminophen without success and was concerned about the risks of additional swelling in her legs and decreased kidney function with NSAIDs. She really did not want an operation. She heard about the risks and potential benefits of taking a low dose of corticosteroids. She asked lots of questions and heard the answers. She started taking prednisone and within a short period of time was able to walk with less difficulty. She did not gain weight. In fact, she had less swelling as she was able to walk farther and stay out of her chair for longer periods of time each day. She tells all her friends how steroids have allowed her to remain in her home.

### Epidural Corticosteroid Injection Therapy

Oral corticosteroids are easy to take, but the disadvantage is they are systemic and affect your entire body. Epidural corticosteroid injections are safe, and complications, infections, or toxicities are rare. Improvement does not occur immediately, and the corticosteroids need days to decrease nerve swelling. Up to a week may be needed before you notice an improvement in leg pain, but improvement lasts for months. Epidural injections should be considered if you do not respond to oral drug therapy and are reluctant to undergo lumbar spine surgery.

The epidural space is inside the spinal canal but outside the covering of the spinal cord (dura). Herniated disc and spinal stenosis compression occur near the epidural space. Epidural corticosteroids have a greater anti-inflammatory effect because the medication comes in direct contract with the inflamed nerve root. The injection is given at the base of the spine near the coccyx (tailbone), or in the lumbar area. The success of the injection can depend on the experience of the health care professional placing the needle. Anesthesiologists and interventional radiologists have extensive experience with epidural injections.

No study has determined the correct number of epidural injections to achieve the maximum effect, but the number should be kept to the minimum. If one injection is adequate for symptom relief, additional injections are not indicated. Epidural injections are limited to a set of three every six months, since no additional benefit is noted with more injections. Also the total dose of corticosteroids in three epidural injections is thought to be safe for a six-month period of exposure. Injections are given no more frequently than every two weeks with the set of three completed over six to eight weeks. People with spinal stenosis can have injections repeated every six months.

One of the misconceptions about epidural corticosteroid injections involves the rapidity of improvement. Some people are disappointed when they do not see immediate reduction in discomfort from sciatica. However, corticosteroids work more slowly than anesthetics. These steroids work by decreasing the inflammation of the disc and nerve, a process that takes time.

In preparation for the injection, you will be asked to stop all medications that are associated with the potential of bleeding, such as aspirin (even small doses), NSAIDs, and blood thinners. This decreases the risk of bleeding. You should also let your doctor know if you are undergoing antibiotic therapy for an infection. The epidural injection may be delayed until the infection is cleared to decrease the possibility of spinal infection. The injection may be given by placement of the needle using body landmarks. In most circumstances, **fluoroscopy** (dynamic X ray images) will be used to identify the spinal level that needs the injection.

### Foraminal Injections

Foraminal stenosis is a condition where the neural foramen at the side of the vertebral body is narrowed. This is a condition similar to spinal stenosis. The patients with foraminal stenosis have leg pain that is more persistent, sitting or standing. The level of narrowing is seen on MRI scans and can be correlated with the location of your symptoms.

A corticosteroid injection directed at the narrow foramen can be effective at relieving pain. The injection is done with radiograph imaging using a fluoroscope. This allows for the needle to be placed in the specific location of narrowing. A series of three injections spaced over weeks is the usual protocol used for these procedures.

## OTHER PAIN THERAPIES

Chronic pain therapy has expanded to a variety of drugs for neurologic conditions. Drugs that are used for seizures (gabapentin, pregabalin) have analgesic benefits. In most circumstances, these drugs are added to NSAIDs and analgesics. Each category of drug is added in sequence to be sure to identify the appearance of any side effects with the newest medicine.

Some antidepressant medicines have pain-relieving properties while others do not. Newer medicines do not always turn out to be better than the older models. Tricyclic antidepressants—Elavil (amitriptyline),

Pamelor (nortriptyline), Tofranil (imipramine)—that are norepinephrine reuptake inhibitors work better for chronic back pain than the newer selective serotonin reuptake inhibitors like Prozac (fluoxetine) or Zoloft (sertraline). The newest generation of antidepressants that are both norepinephrine and serotonin reuptake inhibitors—Cymbalta (duloxetine), Savella (milnacipran)—do demonstrate pain-relieving properties and have been approved for the treatment of pain associated with fibromyalgia.

Also being developed are antibody therapies that inhibit nerve growth factors. These nerve factors are generated in acute and chronic pain states. They inhibit the normal function of nerves. Studies in back pain patients have shown a decrease in pain when infused with these antibodies. The development of this class of antibody will offer a form of pain relief not currently available.

Nonpharmacologic therapies are also an important component of pain relief. This form of therapy includes physical therapy and exercises, which is the subject of the next chapter.

---

### DR. B'S PRESCRIPTION SUMMARY

- Anti-inflammatory drug therapy decreases pain and inflammation and helps keep you functioning.
- Topical anti-inflammatory drugs can be applied to the back for pain relief when oral medicines are contraindicated.
- Muscle relaxants decrease muscle spasms when used in combination with NSAIDs.
- Muscle relaxants do not need to make you too sleepy to work.
- Analgesics—both nonopioid and opioid—relieve pain but do not decrease inflammation.
- Corticosteroids in low doses can be helpful without causing severe side effects.
- Maximizing the beneficial effects of drug therapy is a trial and error process. You may need to try a few different kinds of medications to find the most pain relief with the fewest side effects.
- Spinal injections with corticosteroids are helpful in resolving sciatica secondary to a herniated disc.

# Chapter 10

# Treatment with Exercise and Physical Therapy

EXERCISE AND PHYSICAL THERAPY can be very important to the treatment of low back pain as long as you know when to use them. Exercise can increase motion and improve healing to an area that has been injured. A physical therapist can recommend exercises and similar therapies to improve and maintain the function of your lumbar spine.

A wide range of exercises is available for the treatment and prevention of low back pain. Flexion (bending forward) and extension (bending backward) are the most widely recommended. Choosing the appropriate exercise program is important, because the wrong exercises can make things worse. You may feel comfortable deciding for yourself, or you could be evaluated by a physical therapist.

## WORKING WITH A PHYSICAL THERAPIST

Physical therapy is useful for low back pain if given at the appropriate time. If given too early, you are too "hot"—meaning that pain is so acute that any attempt to improve movement causes increased muscle spasm resulting in marked pain. Exercise can make acute back pain worse if you begin too early in the course of recovery from a back injury, according to a study by the Agency for Healthcare Research and Quality (AHRQ), an organization that published therapy guidelines in 1994. Stretching back muscles or doing strength exercises in the early stages of an episode of acute low back pain can cause greater pain.

The time for exercises is when pain starts to decrease and movement is increasing. You can start with simple flexion and extension exercises without a visit to a physical therapist, but if back pain is not going away and you still can't move any better, then a physical therapist can be helpful to improve function. There are many reasons for completing a course of physical therapy and exercise: to

- Decrease the pain
- Strengthen your muscles
- Stretch your muscles
- Decrease stress to your spinal structures
- Improve fitness to reduce chance of recurrence
- Stabilize your back problem
- Improve your posture
- Improve your mobility

As we age, intervertebral discs are pancakes, not pillows. Therefore, the discs are unable to sustain as many shocks. We must consider new ways to use our back muscles and body position to protect our spine. Physical therapy and exercises help us reach that goal.

No single set of exercise works for all causes of acute and chronic low back pain. In independent studies, flexion and extension exercises are shown to be helpful for chronic low back pain. In a study examining both flexion and extension exercises in the same group of people with low back pain, both sets of exercises were helpful, with flexion exercises resulting in significantly improved front-to-back motion. Before you begin any of these exercises, check with your doctor or health care provider to be sure they are appropriate for you.

### Physical Therapist or Personal Trainer?

One more precaution. Many of my patients have confused the role of a personal trainer with that of a physical therapist. Personal trainers have expertise in exercises to maximize function. The role of these trainers is that of drill sergeant to maximize your exercise to the point of exhaustion. These exercises may be indicated when you are well, but they may put you at risk if your back has not fully healed. A physical therapist works with people who are unable to function in their daily activities because of physical pain. Do not confuse them.

### Physical Therapy Evaluation

An evaluation by a physical therapist is more than the application of heat packs or being given a sheet of exercises. Therapists will review the prescription given to you by your physician. They will take a history of your problem and evaluate your physical capabilities and limitations and try to identify the movements that cause and alleviate your pain. They will use physical means to correct those abnormalities in function. Therapists may use heat or cold modalities, ultrasound, or massage to relieve pain. They will prescribe exercises that will improve back function. The following are some of the exercises they may suggest.

## FLEXION EXERCISES

The mechanism by which exercises produce pain relief is not completely known, but many reasons make common sense. Back and leg pain can come from compression of nerves when enlarged facet joints narrow the neural foramen. Bending forward would open these holes for the nerves and decrease nerve compression. Flexion stretches tighten muscles that move the hip and low back in a backward direction and strengthen abdominal and buttock muscles. In addition, increasing intra-abdominal pressure has the potential of increased support of the lumbar spine. Do not use flexion exercises if you have a herniated disc or if you have leg pain in a seated position.

Flexion exercises are helpful if you have

- Pain in the low back with prolonged standing and relief when you sit
- Pain in the low back when you bend backward and relief when you bend forward
- Spondylolisthesis (the front of your spinal column is not attached to the back of the column)
- Spinal stenosis (leg pain with walking that is relieved with sitting)

Do flexion exercises in the proper sequence—from a resting state to stretching and then to stretching and strengthening. You can use an exercise table or a mat on the floor. Never do flexion exercises with both legs straight. This increases tension in the psoas muscle, in front of the lumbar spine. Increased tension in this muscle increases the pressure in the spinal discs and may increase pain in your back. In fact, doing sit-ups this way can give you a back pain if you don't already have one.

# Acute Relaxation Phase

Figure 10.1. Resting position. Flex your hips with pillows under your knees for fifteen minutes.

Figure 10.2. Resting position. Do it without pillows for fifteen minutes.

Figure 10.3. Back rotation. Keep your shoulders on the table or floor while you turn your pelvis and legs with your knees together. Turn to one side as much as you can tolerate or for one minute. Alternate sides.

# Stretching Phase

Figure 10.4.   Pull your knees up to your chest while raising your pelvis. Hold this for a count of three and relax to the count of six. Begin with one leg at a time and advance to both legs as you improve.

Figure 10.5.   Crossover leg exercise. Place your heel on you opposite knee and pull the bent knee across your body to the opposite shoulder. Hold for a count of three and then relax for the count of six. Alternate legs and do ten repetitions.

Figure 10.6.    Hamstring stretch with knee bent. Bend your knee and flex your hip for a count of three and then relax for a count of six.

Figure 10.7.    Hamstring stretch with straight leg. Hold for three, then relax for six.

Figure 10.8.    Partial sit-up. Bend your knees and put your arms on your chest. Hold for three then relax for a count of six. Repeat this with variation from the easiest to most difficult: arms straight out, arms folded on chest, hands behind head.

Figure 10.9.    Pelvic tilt in standing position. Every hour flatten your low back against a wall with your knees bent. Hold for a count of three every hour. This movement is not only basic to sexual intercourse but is also one of the best ways to stretch the muscles on the back of the spine and strengthen the front ones. The pelvic tilt can be done with a small, nonprovocative motion even in the presence of others. This exercise can be done when sitting, standing, or lying flat. Try it, you'll like it.

## Isometric Back Flexion Exercises

Paul Williams's flexion exercises use motion to improve muscle function as illustrated in figures 10.6 through 10.9. Another form of flexion exercises improves muscle function without any movement. These are isometric exercises—meaning that the muscle contracts but does not move. Use these exercises if even small motions of your back cause pain. Isometrics can strengthen muscles but do not promote flexibility.

Start isometric back flexion exercises by pushing down on your abdominal muscles as if you were forcing a bowel movement. This is the Valsalva maneuver. The same process that works with that bodily function contracts muscles in the abdomen. As you close off your throat and push, your abdominal muscles contract but do not move. Count from five to fifteen as you can tolerate it, then rest. Work up to sets of ten to fifteen repetitions three to four times a day.

The next set of exercises involves the buttocks. Squeeze your cheeks (the gluteus muscles) together. Count between five to fifteen, then rest. If you are coordinated, try a Valsalva maneuver and cheek squeeze together. The result of these two actions is a sustained pelvic tilt with tightened buttock muscles. These exercises strengthen the flexor muscles and give you greater stability.

## EXTENSION EXERCISES

In contrast to Paul Williams's flexion exercises, Robin McKenzie, a physical therapist from New Zealand, proposed extension exercises as a means to decrease pain. He suggested that leg pain came from a disc herniation pressing on a spinal nerve and by bending backward you could force the ruptured part of the disc back to its normal location. However, this method has not proven effective in relieving sciatica. Nerve compression causes leg numbness, not pain. Nerve inflammation causes sciatic pain. (Neither Williams's nor McKenzie's exercise methods acutely change inflammation in an irritated spinal nerve.)

The purpose of extension exercises is to strengthen the muscles along the spine and to improve your endurance and spinal mobility, and also to increase the stamina of the lumbar spine, center the gel—or cushion—inside the disc, and decrease your risk of reinjury.

Extension exercises are helpful if you have

- Pain in the low back with prolonged sitting or driving
- Pain in the low back with bending forward
- Pain in the low back rising from a chair
- Pain in the leg that is increased with sitting
- Relief with lying flat
- Relief with walking

Extension exercises should follow a progression during the early phase of low back pain.

### Acute Relaxation Phase

Figure 10.10.    Lie facedown with pillows under you abdomen. Add more pillows as you can tolerate it. Do this for fifteen minutes.

# Stretching Phase

Figure 10.11. Prop yourself up on bent elbows and hold for three then relax to a count of six.

Figure 10.12. Place your hands on your low back and bend backward. Hold for three then relax to a count of six. Repeat this hourly.

Figure 10.13. Prop yourself up on outstretched arms (like a push-up movement). Hold for ten and do ten repetitions.

## Strengthening Phase

Figure 10.14.   Raise your head and legs off the floor as much as you can tolerate. Hold this position for a count of three and then relax to a count of six.

Figure 10.15.   Now raise yourself up and maintain a normal seated posture with a curved back.

### Variations

A variation to extension strengthening exercises can be tried when you are "on all fours." Attempt this only after your back pain has begun to improve. Stretch out your arm and the opposite leg parallel to the floor. Hold this position for a count of two and then return your arm and leg to the floor. Do the same motion with the opposite arm and leg. Try to increase repetitions in the Comfort Zone as you can tolerate them. You should try for a goal of ten to fifteen lifts.

After two weeks of doing these flexion and extension exercises, you can add another set of exercises to your routine.

Figure 10.16. Lateral bending in the standing position. Put your hand on opposite side of your head with the other arm sliding down your leg. Hold for a count of ten and repeat every hour.

Figure 10.17. Lying on your side, hold your top leg straight and move it behind you. Hold for three then relax for six.

Figure 10.18. Lying on your side, raise your leg away from your body. Hold for three then relax for six.

Figure 10.19.  Lying on your side, lift your head and legs off the bed. Hold for
three then relax for six.

## THE "C" AND "S" CURVES

Sometimes muscles are in so much spasm that the spine is bent into
a "C" or an "S." Not everyone has spasm to this degree, but there's
something that can help you find out if you do. An experienced physical therapist, Tom Welsh, taught me that people could determine the
exercises that would help their back curve. Here are his suggestions.
First, decide which letter of the alphabet, "C" or "S," best fits your
shape. Stand in front of a full-length mirror and compare the height of
your shoulders and hips.

Figure 10.20.  Right "C" curve—the left
shoulder and right hip are higher.

Figure 10.21.  Left "C" curve—the right
shoulder and left hip are higher.

Heal Your Back

Figure 10.22. Front "S" curve—the left shoulder and left hip are higher.

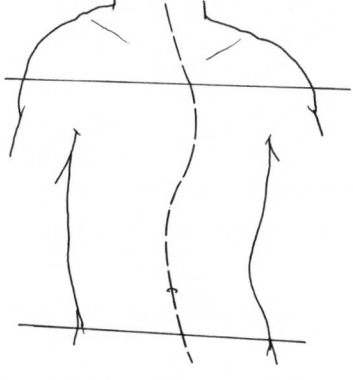

Figure 10.23. Backward "S" curve—the right shoulder and right hip are higher.

Use your right and left arms or legs depending on the type of curve you have. Do these exercises on the floor or in bed. These exercises improve flexibility but also stabilize the spine, which improves function and decreases pain.

Figure 10. 24. Exercise 1—Lie on your stomach. Raise a straight leg a few inches off the bed and overstretch it downward. Hold for a count of three. Repeat ten times. (Right "C" and Front "S"—left leg; Left "C" and Backward "S"—right leg.)

Figure 10.25. Exercise 2—Lie on your back. Bend your knees. Raise a bent knee and push your hand against the knee with equal resistance. At the same time pull your opposite knee toward your chest. Hold for a count of three. Repeat ten times. (Right "C" and Front "S"—raise right knee and pull left knee; Left "C" and Backward "S"—raise left knee and pull right knee.)

Figure 10.26. Exercise 3—Lie on your side. Align your legs with your body. Raise the top leg up and down twelve to eighteen inches. Repeat twenty-five times (Right "C" and Front "S"—left side down, right leg raises; Left "C" and Backward "S"—right side down, left leg raises.)

Figure 10.27. Exercise 4—Lie on your back. Bend your knees and keep your knees and heels together. Roll both knees to the side. Hold for a count of twenty. Tighten your stomach muscles and keep them tight while you roll your knees back to the center. Repeat three times. (Right "C"—roll right; Left "C"—roll left.)

Figure 10.28.    Exercise 5—Lie on your back. Bend your knees and keep your knees and heels together. Put a pillow under your shoulder and upper back. Roll both knees to the side with the pillow. Hold for a count of twenty. Tighten your stomach muscles and keep them tight while you roll your knees back to the center. Repeat three times. (Front "S"—pillow left shoulder, roll left; Backward "S"—pillow right shoulder, roll right.)

Figure 10.29.    Exercise 6—Get down on your hands and knees. Align your knees with your hips and your hands with your shoulders. Raise your knee up and down one to two inches. Repeat twenty-five times. (Right "C" and Backward "S"—raise left knee; Left "C" and Front "S"—raise right knee.)

Figure 10.30.    Exercise 7—Lie on your stomach. Keep your arms at your sides. Raise your chest and shoulders up and down and arch your back. Repeat this twenty-five times at a rapid pace. (All curves.)

## TRANSCUTANEOUS ELECTRICAL NERVE STIMULATION (TENS)

Physical therapists sometimes use TENS therapy with surface electrodes applied to the skin. (Electrodes can be implanted directly on a nerve or sensory column of the spinal cord but only by a neurosurgeon.)

TENS works by stimulating high-speed nerve fibers that block the slower speed pain fibers. Different forms of electrical signals are needed to stimulate nerve fibers. The settings on the TENS machine (transcutaneous stimulator) are modified to find the correct wave pulse that works best for you.

Once the appropriate setting is reached, you will feel a tingling sensation in the stimulated area. The sensation should not cause an unpleasant sensation or muscle contracture. Therapy sessions should last for a minimum of thirty minutes to determine if therapy has benefit. The onset of pain relief can be measured from minutes to hours. The average time is twenty minutes. The duration of pain relief is variable. Some people have had relief lasting days to weeks from a short course of therapy. TENS does not work for everyone.

## IONTOPHORESIS: ANOTHER FORM OF "INJECTION" THERAPY

Iontophoresis is a machine that uses direct electrical current from a 9-volt battery to transfer a medicine across a body surface without the need for an injection. Local anesthetics and soluble corticosteroids are the medicines most frequently given by iontophoresis. The medicine is injected into a pad that is placed over the painful area. The treatment takes about twenty minutes to complete. The frequency of treatments corresponds to the pain relief. The treatment cannot be repeated too frequently because of the buildup of corticosteroids. However, treatments can be given intermittently, over extended periods of time. On occasion, iontophoresis delivers local pain relief that can have significant effects on overall function.

A fifty-eight-year-old man's hobby was riding motorcycles. Over the past two years, his riding had decreased because he would experience right buttock pain that would increase over time. He had tried medicines but had an NSAID sensitivity that prevented his use of NSAIDs and COX-2 medications. He had tried local injections in the past but had none recently. He had developed atrial fibrillation, a fluttering of the heart that required taking blood thinners on a daily basis. He would bleed excessively with any injections. He was depressed because he could not get back out on his bike. My suggestion was that he try iontophoresis over his painful buttock area. The therapy was helpful, and pain relief lasted for an extended period of time. He used the therapy intermittently when he had a return of pain and he was going to ride his motorcycle.

Iontophoresis can be used for pain in other superficial locations. This therapy is applied by physical therapists with a prescription from a physician for the therapy and the medication. Some physicians also offer the therapy in their offices.

### GETTING IN THE WATER

Another place to do exercises is in the water. The exercises that you find difficult to do on land may be much easier to complete when you are floating in the water. Additional benefit may be gained if the pool is heated. Water exercises can help in the following ways:

- Provides balanced strengthening of flexion and extension muscles through force of resistance of the water
- Offers support to decrease the risk of injury from falling
- Allows for a greater range of motion and coordination through muscle relaxation
- Allows for the opportunity to increase aerobic and anaerobic fitness

Exercises in the pool should be done at a pace that is comfortable. You can start with walking normally in a straight line, swinging your arms. As you progress, you may do lateral bends both right and left without twisting. As you strengthen you can add leg kicks. This exercise is completed by standing in the pool, holding on to one of the sides. You raise the leg opposite to the arm holding the side of the pool. You raise the straight leg forward as is comfortable, and then behind, repeating these movements several times. You then repeat with the other leg.

A water or aquatics program can help everyone but can be particularly helpful for my obese patients. Obesity may not cause back pain but it is more difficult to relieve it if you are overweight. My patients tell me that they would love to do land exercises but have too much difficulty completing them. Getting these patients into the water can make all the difference.

## Water Baby Wanda

Wanda is a forty-eight-year-old woman who developed back pain after lifting boxes while moving her mother out of her home. She was overweight and had been on a number of diets without much benefit. She had tried to exercise but found that walking at lunchtime was difficult and hurt her knees if she went too far. She was treated with an NSAID medicine and as she improved was told to start flexion exercises. She returned two weeks later with only a minimal amount of discomfort but with concern that she had not completed her exercises. She wanted to know if she could do the exercises in some other fashion. I told her about a pool program organized by the local Arthritis Foundation. About a month later, Wanda returned with no pain and about five pounds lighter. She had become a "water baby." She loved the water aquatics program. She had started slowly just walking in the water and doing leg lifts. As she felt more comfortable she did more of the back and leg exercises. Her back felt better as did her knee.

Remember the water if land exercises seem too difficult.

A variety of physical therapy methods are available to a therapist to help your problem. These include manual resistance methods, core stabilization, neuromobilization techniques, and manipulation of soft tissues to name a few. Your therapist will choose the best technique for your problem and will also educate you with the physical means to maintain your improvement. Become an "exercise nut." If you do your exercises, the chances of needing to see your doctor about back pain will be decreased significantly.

Exercises are only as good as the frequency with which they are done. I have given many printed and illustrated exercise directions to patients who promise that they will do their exercises regularly. They return a bit sheepish admitting that they had no time in their schedules for what they knew would be helpful to their condition.

The best successes I have had are with people who followed their exercise routine on a regular basis. They stopped their medicines and remained functional even though at times the beneficial response was delayed.

## The "Religious" Cabinetmaker

A forty-eight-year-old cabinetmaker developed back pain after standing in an extended posture for a number of hours while installing a set of heavy cabinets. He developed severe muscle spasm and increased back pain with extending his spine. I gave him an NSAID and a muscle relaxant for relief of his symptoms. Then I educated him about the importance of flexion exercises and the danger of bending backward. He gradually improved, and within one month he was back at work building and installing cabinets. He could not stop his medicines without developing a return of his back pain. He wanted to stop his medicines but had to continue to work. I told him to continue to do his exercises on a regular basis. He did his exercises religiously. After a year, he did not need his muscle relaxant. He was about ready to stop his NSAID when he stopped exercising. He had a relapse of his pain. He returned to his exercises and within the next year was able to stop all his medicine. Currently, he is building cabinets, doing his exercises, and staying off medicines. Only after he became "religious" with his exercises did his back pain remain controlled.

Exercises do make a difference. A flexible and strong lower back is an anchor to a number of our daily activities. If you put in the work, you will gain the benefit.

## DR. B'S PRESCRIPTION SUMMARY

- Exercises and physical therapy play a greater role during the later healing phase of healing acute low back pain.
- No one type of exercise program fits all types of back pain, but flexion (bending forward) and extension (bending backward) exercises are most widely recommended by doctors and physical therapists.
- Exercises are also important if you have chronic low back pain because they will stretch and strengthen your back muscles and help improve mobility and reduce pain.
- Exercises are most effective when you do them regularly.
- A physical trainer is not the same as a physical therapist.
- Steroids can be delivered through the skin to superficial structures without a needle with electrical current from a battery (iontophoresis).
- Get in the water. Aquatic exercises can be helpful to you no matter what your size or physical capabilities.
- Aerobic exercise through walking on land or in the pool is a good exercise to improve stamina and strength of back muscles. Aerobic exercise also has other general health benefits.

# Chapter 11

# Complementary Therapies

CULTURES THROUGHOUT THE WORLD have used healing techniques that today fall into the category of complementary therapy. Some of these therapies were accepted in India and China, for example, well before scientific methods became available to prove their effectiveness for improving certain medical conditions. We still do not know the mechanism of action for some complementary therapies, and some physicians and others believe the benefits are largely a **placebo** effect. But whatever the effect, more attention is being paid in medical schools and by practicing physicians. For instance, some conventional doctors have actually learned how to give acupuncture treatments.

In 1997 an estimated 629 million visits were made to practitioners of complementary therapies, while only 388 million were made to primary care physicians. Four of ten Americans use complementary therapies to some extent. The National Institutes of Health recognized the utilization of these therapies by the public and established the National Center for Complementary and Alternative Medicine in 1998 to study these methods.

Low back pain sufferers are frequent visitors to practitioners of complementary medicine such as chiropractors, acupuncturists, and bodywork specialists. Complementary therapies seem most popular among those who cannot find satisfaction with conventional therapies or who have a condition that is unpredictable—such as low back pain. Such therapies are also considered relatively risk-free and cheaper than conventional medicine. Without choosing well, however, none of these considerations are true.

The term "complementary medicine" implies that such therapies are used in concert with conventional therapies for low back pain, while the term "alternative" therapy suggests that these therapies are mutually exclusive, which is not the case. However, I view complementary methods as passive therapies, which, for the most part, are done to back pain patients. This is particularly true of chiropractic, osteopathic, and bodywork therapies. I prefer active therapies such as education about self-directed exercise regimens that enable you to take control of your condition.

You may seek complementary therapies based on a friend's recommendation, an advertisement, or past experience. Regardless of the reason, tell your doctor about every vitamin, natural supplement, special diet, exercise, or manual therapy you are using. Your physician may have experience with complementary practitioners and, therefore, can offer recommendations.

These therapies are here to stay. Some can help your back pain, but use them wisely and only to

- Enhance the effects of conventional therapies
- Improve your outlook
- Ease symptoms of chronic pain, stress, and anxiety

In general, complementary therapies cannot

- Cure any illness
- Improve acute illnesses rapidly
- Replace conventional therapies

## MANUAL MANIPULATION

A prominent group of complementary therapists, including chiropractors, osteopaths, and massage therapists, believe that the natural healing processes of the body are facilitated through manipulation and movement of soft tissues and repositioning of body parts. They believe their treatments remove blockages and result in improved function by moving the spine back to its normal position. Some disciplines believe that a variety of illnesses can be treated through this manipulation of the musculoskeletal system, but this remains controversial.

# Chiropractic Manipulation

Chiropractic manipulation seems to be most effective for acute low back pain of short duration, usually a month or less. Good candidates for this therapy are younger individuals between the ages of twenty and fifty. Some people improve with the first session; others require several treatments. If a month of therapy has passed without improvement, chiropractic treatment will not help you.

Studies show the benefit of chiropractic manipulation for low back pain without sciatica, but these benefits are short term, and chronic low back pain does not appear to benefit from chiropractic therapy. Occasionally, chiropractic adjustment may encourage movement in those with limited motion and chronic back pain.

In certain situations, manipulation can have serious effects on your health. For example, it is not recommended for people with sciatica (leg pain). Adjustments may make a disc herniation worse, causing loss of strength or loss of bladder and rectal function.

Older people should be especially cautious about chiropractic adjustment if they have osteoporosis or small fractures in a vertebra. Adjustments will not be helpful if you have spinal stenosis associated with some back but more leg pain with walking. There is added risk if you are taking blood-thinning medication. Some of the chiropractic adjustments can cause bleeding. If you have one of these conditions, consult with a medical doctor before undergoing chiropractic manipulation because the treatment may not be safe for you.

The premise of chiropractic therapy is that misaligned vertebrae (**subluxations**) cause most illness by blocking the nervous system and interfering with natural healing. Adjusting the spine to its natural position reverses this process, resulting in a cure. Chiropractors make adjustments with gentle pressures or more forceful thrusts to the spine. Sometimes this generates a popping sound like cracking knuckles. Sudden force on the joint forms negative atmospheric pressure, a vacuum in the joint. The popping sound is created by the generation of a bubble of nitrogen gas that is moved rapidly in the joint. The popping sound of the spine does not cause arthritis, just like cracking your knuckles does not cause arthritis. Chiropractic adjustments and movement should be painless. Physical therapists also use manipulation to maximize motion of musculoskeletal structures, but they use more gradual motions to achieve the same outcome.

Scott, a thirty-four-year-old accountant, had surgery for a herniated disc. His leg pain improved but then recurred in six months and radiated down to the back of his buttock. Medication helped, but Scott wanted to decrease his need. He had six treatments with a chiropractor and had significant improvement in his back and thigh pain. This treatment allowed him to reduce his NSAID use to every other day—but he was not pain-free.

### Choosing a Chiropractor

Chiropractors may use manipulation alone or in combination with other complementary therapies. "Straight" chiropractors do only spinal manipulation; "mixers" use a variety of therapies—including nutritional supplements, homeopathic remedies, and acupuncture—to achieve balance in the nervous system. They often take X rays before beginning manipulation therapy. Many such X rays demonstrate slight curvatures, which may then be suggested as the cause of pain. However, the significance of these curvatures is questionable, because many people without back pain show similar degrees of curvature on spine X rays. Question the need for X rays before you begin treatment with a chiropractor, and see a medical doctor if you suspect any serious illness is causing your pain.

Questions need to be raised about "maintenance therapy" that is prescribed for months or years. Chronic manipulations of the spine may cause more pain than they relieve. You should learn the exercises to maintain your improvement.

Make sure you choose a good chiropractor. While chiropractic treatment for low back pain is unlikely to harm you, injury is more likely if the practitioner has little understanding of the musculoskeletal system and the effects of adjustments on the lumbar spine.

You will know if a chiropractor is good if he or she

- Takes time to listen to your problem
- Does not require X rays for treatment of acute low back pain
- Provides a time frame for the course of therapy
- Treats only musculoskeletal disorders
- Lets you pay for one visit at a time
- Is willing to refer to a medical doctor if therapy is ineffective

Many chiropractors are affiliated with hospitals, health maintenance organizations, and large group practices, and you may also find a referral from friends and family. Just be sure to ask questions that provide information about the issues raised above.

## Osteopathic Manipulation

Dr. Andrew Taylor Still developed the philosophy of osteopathic medicine because he believed in a unifying principle between body structure and function in health and disease. Still also believed physicians overlooked the body's ability to heal itself, a philosophy that was not accepted by allopathic (conventional) physicians in the late 1800s. Dr. Still started his own school of osteopathic medicine in 1892, and osteopathic schools soon were established throughout the United States. Today, the curriculum studied by osteopathic physicians (D.O.'s) and allopathic physicians (M.D.'s) is quite similar, but osteopaths also specialize in how disordered physical structures affect function. Allopathic and osteopathic physicians are licensed with similar rights and privileges.

The osteopathic physician observes abnormalities in structure, such as muscle spasm, restriction of motion, or sensitivity to palpation. The spine is considered the primary area of dysfunction because of its proximity to the autonomic nervous system, which monitors all the basic functions of the body. Osteopathic manipulation of the spine and other structures restores normal body mechanics and function, thereby restoring balance in the organ systems, including the nervous system. Improved function also results in improved blood flow. Osteopathic treatment may involve manipulation alone, a combination of manipulation and other complementary therapies, or drug therapy.

A variety of osteopathic techniques are available for the treatment of low back pain. Myofascial release, strain and counterstrain, cranial techniques (gentle manipulation of the head and spine), and manipulation with impulse (greater force) are some of the techniques that may be useful. Osteopathic manipulation has been shown to decrease back pain, but the benefit may be limited to a few weeks.

There are over fifty thousand osteopathic physicians in the United States, licensed through individual states; many belong to the American Osteopathic Association. Some D.O.'s deliver only allopathic care; some D.O.'s offer only certain forms of manipulation; and still others offer a wide variety of complementary therapies, too. Let your outlook for your back problem guide you in deciding if a D.O. offers therapy that will be helpful to you. And be sure to tell your osteopath if spinal manipulation increases your pain.

## MASSAGE AND OTHER BODYWORK TECHNIQUES

The ancient Greek physician Hippocrates, the "father of medicine," believed that massage freed nutritive fluids to flow to the body's organs. The Romans further developed massage practices as part of their healing system. Eastern cultures in India and China have also developed massage techniques and promoted their benefits. Today we have various massage styles, mostly based on Eastern or Western techniques.

Western massage, such as Swedish massage, can relax tense muscles to improve range of motion, remove stress, and increase energy. The pressure on muscles brings a different sensation into the tissues and relieves pain. Chinese and Japanese forms of massage, such as shiatsu, improve the flow of energy (**qi**) through the body's energy channels (meridians). Pressure on acupuncture points releases blocked qi and restores the body's natural balance.

### Reflexology

Reflexologists believe that the organs of the body have representations on different areas of the feet, hands, and ears. Thus, massaging reflex points on the feet and hands can influence vital organs in a distant location. The spinal column is located along the instep of the foot, for example. The lumbar spine is found in a vertical orientation near the ankle bone. Treatment of the lower back and sacrum includes pressure with a rocking motion over the back, lateral quadrant of the heel. Treatment of the lumbar spine uses pressure over the instep near the heel bone with upward movement toward the ankle. The spine is also represented along the ear rim, as well as the hand. By placing pressure on the reflex points, particularly in the feet, energy is released in the affected area, resulting in relaxation and pain relief.

### Craniosacral Massage

This massage tries to balance the system that connects the skull (cranio) with the base of the spine (sacrum). Light touch is placed on the skull to balance muscle tension, and the sacrum may also be manipulated. This is gentle massage, with little risk of damaging underlying tissues.

### Rolfing/Structural Integration

The theory behind rolfing, named for Ida Rolf, Ph.D., is that thickened fascia (the membrane covering your muscles) results from accumulated physical imbalances related to specific injuries, such as a hip strain. Connective tissue may shorten around the injury, which adds to unbalanced movements and postures. Rolfing is essentially a deep tissue massage technique involving vigorous movement to loosen adhesions of connective tissues covering these injuries. The technique can be painful as the tensions in joints, ligaments, and muscles are released. The therapy is given in ten one-hour weekly sessions.

### How to Choose the Best Bodywork for You

Bodywork refers to a group of manual therapies that promote improved body mechanics and decreased stress. Get the most out of your bodywork technique by planning before your session in the following ways:

- Identify the goals of the technique you choose.
- Visit only an experienced practitioner.
- Tell the practitioner about your concerns.
- Rest after your session to enjoy its benefits.
- Talk with your therapist about any necessary preparation.

Massage techniques may use a light touch or a more vigorous stretching of muscles, so decide which type of massage you would most enjoy. Experienced bodywork therapists deliver the best sessions, so find a practitioner who knows the particulars of your condition and the useful techniques for your specific problem. Contact organizations that certify massage therapists or the licensing board of your state to determine the status of the practitioner you are considering. In addition, gather recommendations from other health professionals or the practitioner's patients.

## ACUPUNCTURE

Acupuncture is based upon the Chinese theory that energy pathways, called meridians, carry the body's energy, which is known as qi or chi. Illness causes an imbalance in the flow of qi in the twelve primary meridians. Stimulation of specific points along the meridians can correct the flow of qi to optimize health or block pain. It also relieves pain through the release of endorphins. More than one million Americans use acupuncture on an ongoing basis, many of them because of musculoskeletal problems.

Traditional acupuncture uses thin needles at the 360 specific points along the meridians to rebalance the flow of energy. Between five and fifteen thin, flexible, solid, sterile needles are inserted from a mere fraction of an inch to four inches deep. As the needles are inserted, you may feel a range of sensations from a light needle prick to tingling, warmth, or pinching. The needles are left in place from five to sixty minutes (twenty minutes is about the average). It may take a course of ten treatments to obtain maximum benefit, and you may need follow-up treatments, usually every few months, to maintain normal energy balance. In addition to needles, or in place of needles, practitioners may use heat, pressure, friction, suction, or electrical current connected to needles on acupuncture points. These may produce similar effects.

When a licensed practitioner does it, acupuncture has a good safety record. However, possible complications include infections (AIDS or hepatitis) if unsterile needles are used, organ punctures, dermatitis, and local bleeding. Make sure your therapist uses sterile disposable needles that are used only once so there is no chance of infection.

Acupuncture is an example of a complementary therapy that supplements the effectiveness of other treatments for chronic pain, including medications and physical therapy. As yet, we do not have good data on the frequency of a positive response to acupuncture treatments. It is worthwhile to try acupuncture if all other therapies have been tried but are not fully effective. Acupuncture should also be considered if toxic side effects prevent the use of medications.

A disadvantage is that the passive, time-consuming procedure is also relatively expensive since it is not yet universally covered by medical insurance, including Medicare.

### Ear Acupuncture

Auriculotherapy is acupuncture of the outer ear. The theory is that the upside-down human body is represented on our ears. Tenderness over parts of the ear corresponds to areas of the body that have been injured. Electrical stimulation of the ear has been reported to increase spinal fluid endorphin levels, our natural opioid chemicals. Many individuals report warmth and other sensations in distant parts of the body with ear stimulation. Acupuncture of the ear is worth a chance to enhance the benefits of other therapies that have not been adequately effective in controlling pain.

## YOGA AND OTHER BODY, MIND, AND SPIRIT TECHNIQUES

Currently popular in the West, yoga has its origin in Indian culture as part of the Ayurvedic form of therapy. The Sanskrit word "yoga" comes from the root *yug*, which means to join. Yoga is a philosophy of life that promotes awareness of the unity of the body, mind, and spirit. Patanjali, an Indian teacher, wrote about the principles of yoga thousands of years ago.

The postures (asanas) and breathing techniques (pranayama) closely associated with yoga in the Western world are means to increase physical strength and stamina needed for meditation. The harmony between physical and mental states brings greater self-awareness and health. In this context, yoga is both preventive and curative for ailments of the body, mind, and spirit.

In Western cultures, yoga postures have become the means to achieve better health, with a lesser emphasis on the mental aspect of meditation and self-realization. Yoga comes in many varieties. Most Westerners know the form called hatha yoga, combining *ha* for "sun," and *tha*, meaning "moon." Hatha yoga is the yoga of activity and is a disciplined system of gentle stretches and balancing exercises. Asanas, if done correctly, affect all the organs of the body. Postures are adjusted so that alignments are correct for the bones, joints, and organs. This proper alignment allows for the ideal function of the body.

The restorative powers of yoga to treat the kind of difficulties associated with back pain would seem an ideal fit. Many people who have learned the yoga postures report improvement in their pain and decreased stress.

### The Stressed-Out Teacher

Alice, a forty-five-year-old elementary school teacher, had low back pain for two years. She could not remember what brought her pain on, but it was a real inconvenience because she had two children and a demanding job. Between her lesson plans and driving her children around to one event or another, she rarely took time to take care of her back, except when the pain became excruciating. Alice would take over-the-counter drugs until the pain lessened, and then she'd quit. She had no time for exercise, and she drank excessive amounts of caffeine during the day, which led to difficulty going to sleep at night.

This stressed-out teacher had many problems, one of which was her back. Eliminating the caffeine was only one of my suggestions, and she began taking an NSAID and started some simple stretching exercises. Her back improved, but she remained anxious and stressed. Alice told me that a friend of hers found yoga helpful for back problems and I encouraged her to go, not only to improve flexibility, but also to benefit from yoga's stress-relieving qualities.

After two years of participating in yoga exercise, Alice has less back discomfort and takes less medication. Equally important, she is much calmer, even though she still has responsibility for many children. Through yoga, Alice has learned to cope with her many stresses and she believes it has made a significant difference in the quality of her life.

Ideally, yoga should be done daily, and periodic classes allow for reinforcement of maintaining correct postures. Many exercise programs recommend rest days in between sessions, but yoga does not entail the kind of muscle strain and strenuous activity that makes rest necessary.

Under the guidance of an experienced teacher, you are at little risk of damage from exercises done correctly. Programs that build from the most safe and simple postures seem most appropriate. If a posture hurts, do not do it.

Choosing a teacher can be challenging. You don't need a license to teach yoga, and the philosophy of the teacher structures the class content and emphasis. Observe a class to determine if its objectives meet your needs. Then show illustrations of yoga postures to your physician and ask if any may be harmful to you.

### "Hot" Yoga

Some of my back pain patients have sung the praises of "hot" or Bikram yoga. This form of yoga uses a ninety-minute class, with twenty-six poses, and two breathing exercises in a room heated to 105 degrees Fahrenheit with 40 percent humidity. This form of yoga is not for the fainthearted. Almost all of my patients who have participated in these classes have been younger. Beginners experience dizziness and nausea. It is difficult to complete a full session. For those who have, they describe a flexibility and reinvigoration that is not the same with regular yoga classes.

### Tai Chi

Tai chi is an ancient Chinese practice that gently moves the body through a number of slow, continuous, flowing postures. Unlike the martial arts, tai chi involves no impact or jarring motions. A session may last from twenty to sixty minutes and promotes deep breathing, balance, and stress reduction. There are five distinct styles of tai chi; some do not require deep knee bending and would be ideal for those with back pain and knee arthritis.

Tai chi has been proven to be effective in improving musculoskeletal function. In a study of 215 people over age seventy, tai chi decreased their risk of falling compared to the same age groups taught balance exercises and behavior modification. These people also had lower blood pressure and improved hand strength. Tai chi may help back pain by improving relaxation and regaining flexibility.

Tai chi is best learned from a teacher. It helps if the teacher has some appreciation of back pain and has had experience with students with this problem. Exercises should be done every day even for short periods of time. Exertion is not part of the process. Relaxation and stress reduction are part of the mental component of tai chi. Do not overlook it.

### Qi Gong

Qi gong is older than tai chi. Qi gong started in China over three thousand years ago. Like tai chi, qi gong uses slow graceful movements and controlled breathing to promote the movement of qi through the body. In general, the movements are fewer and less graceful than tai chi. Each movement is separate and held for seconds at a time. Some movements only use the arms and spare the rest of the body. The importance of the movements is to mobilize your qi to be less stressed, depressed, and more functional.

### The Pilates Method

Joseph Pilates was a fitness trainer in Germany who emigrated to the United States in 1926. He developed "centrology," a system that incorporates the science and art of coordinated body-mind-spirit development through natural movements under strict control of the will. This method encompasses elements of Western and Eastern philosophy regarding the importance of motion and strength in the setting of inner calm and relaxation. Initially, Pilates was particularly popular with dancers like Martha Graham. More recently, with a growth in the number of Pilates studios and instructors, it has gained greater acceptance by the general public.

The program includes over five hundred different exercises designed to increase balance, flexibility, and strength by building more efficient muscles. Exercises are performed on a mat, a wall, or Pilates apparatus including springs, barrels, and chairs. The program concentrates on strengthening abdominal, buttock, and spinal muscles. According to Sean Gallagher and Romana Kryzanowska, instructors of the Pilates Method, the six basic principles are concentration to movement, control of movement by the mind, strengthening the center of the body, flowing movement, precision, and proper breathing. Specific exercises are recommended for those with back pain.

A key to success with the Pilates Method is a well-trained and experienced teacher. Observation by an instructor can assure that your technique is correct. The number of teachers has grown but is limited to major cities in the United States and a few foreign countries. The website for instructors has updated information about instructors and their studios. Many of the exercises can be done on a mat without the use of an apparatus. Books and videos of the exercises are available for those who wish to try the conditioning program on their own. The potential harm from Pilates exercises is doing them incorrectly. Tensions placed across the low back have the potential to aggravate structures like narrowed disc spaces. Listen to what your body is telling you. Modify your program if pain is increased.

## MIND-BODY THERAPIES

Another form of complementary therapy is based upon the interaction between chronic pain and disease and psychological stress. Pain, when associated with a change in personality and thinking, may persist even after the original injury has healed. Negative emotions heighten pain and anxiety and increase muscle tension, and may lead to or exacerbate depression. Improving your emotional state has a beneficial effect on your physical status. Mind-body therapies include biofeedback, hypnosis, cognitive-behavioral therapy, relaxation techniques, stress reduction, meditation, and guided imagery.

The therapies discussed below may increase your sense of self-control and accomplishment, but we do not all benefit from the same therapy. Investigate the techniques that appeal to you, and if one doesn't help, try another. These therapies have few side effects and are inexpensive, but they require time and effort. They may be used in combination with other therapies such as medications.

## Biofeedback

Electronic monitors help you learn how to use your mind to control other body functions. Back pain often increases muscle tension, and surface electromyographs (EMGs) can detect electrical signals generated by your muscles. The intensity of these signals is shown on a computer screen. The biofeedback practitioner teaches you how to use your mind to decrease the intensity of the muscle tension, which is shown on the computer as fewer signals. As you become more expert at the technique, you no longer need the EMG to confirm muscle relaxation, and you can do the technique any time without the equipment.

The key to success with biofeedback is persistence, because you need time to learn the technique. The advantages of biofeedback include lack of side effects and its portability—it travels wherever you go.

## Hypnosis

Hypnosis is an altered state of awareness that allows you to narrow your attention and exclude extraneous stimulation. In the hypnotic state your intense concentration places your attention between wakefulness and deep sleep, to promote deep relaxation. In addition, pain may be decreased directly or may be transferred to another part of the body, or the type or quality of the pain may change to a sense of numbness or tingling. Initially, a hypnotherapist induces a hypnotic state, but you can learn techniques to hypnotize yourself and attain a trance.

Some psychiatrists utilize hypnosis as part of therapy, but other practitioners are not licensed. Before undergoing a session, inquire about the hypnotherapist's experience. Understand, too, that while you're suggestible in a hypnotic trance, you will not do anything that goes against your wishes. In other words, you remain in control.

## Visualization

Visualization coaxes you to imagine your desired outcome. After relaxing with breathing exercises or progressive relaxation, focus your mind on specific sensations that are meaningful to you. To achieve a degree of pain relief, you might create an image of your muscle being its normal length or an image of the painful part or spot being swept away.

Jim, sixty-three, had left-sided low back pain and numbness in his foot while walking. He also had extensive practice in the martial arts and as a judo expert; he spent many hours focusing his thoughts on controlling his body as he performed judo. Jim's X rays indicated a narrowed neural foramen pressing on a nerve. Celebrex and stretching exercises improved his symptoms. One day, he told me about his visualization technique, which he believed helped relieve his pain. After completing breathing exercises, he focused his thoughts at the joint that had closed around his nerve. He visualized this joint opening up and relieving the pressure on his nerve. When his relaxation period was over, he realized that he could walk farther with less discomfort. His positive thoughts had helped bring about a good outcome, but he also understood that his visualization technique offered temporary relief, and he scheduled an MRI to determine the extent of his nerve compression.

Like relaxation techniques, visualization has no side effects and it is certainly cost-effective. Tapes are available to help you learn these techniques, and some provide guided visualization. In order to benefit from visualization you must decide if you believe that a mental function can have an effect on physical symptoms.

### Cognitive Behavioral Therapy

Cognitive behavioral therapy (CBT) utilizes psychological techniques to improve the coping skills of individuals who have chronic pain, including back pain. The program does not eliminate pain but decreases recurrences and reduces their impact. Some of the interventional strategies include fear reduction, coping strategies, stress management, and problem solving. CBT gives you the tools to make your life better. Therapy is usually offered by a psychologist who is trained in these techniques. In locations where CBT therapists are unavailable, some of the techniques can be learned through the use of the Internet. An example of an Internet website that offers some of the tools of CBT is www.knowfibro.com. Although this site is directed at fibromyalgia patients, it contains a tool that deals with stress management, sleep hygiene, and coping skills that can help with your back pain. Recent studies have shown that CBT can be very effective in reducing pain and disability in chronic back pain patients. Of particular interest is the durability of the therapy to last twelve months or longer after the sessions are completed. This duration of benefit is noteworthy and makes CBT particularly useful as a treatment for chronic low back pain.

## MEDITATION AND RELAXATION

Meditation is another technique that focuses the mind on a thought or sensation, and although we tend to associate meditation with Eastern philosophies and religion, the positive effects do not require religious or spiritual orientation. Focusing your mind on a single word or phrase can elicit the benefits of the relaxation response. Over time, silent repetition of a word or phrase can result in a change in consciousness. One of my patients explained the process by saying that meditation is not about falling asleep, but rather, is a silent concentration on thoughts, emotions, and sensations.

To meditate, you need a quiet place without distractions and a sitting posture that is comfortable and stable. (The crossed-legged lotus position is not necessary.) Meditation starts with deep breathing while focusing your thoughts on a meaningful word, phrase, or object. As every beginner knows, your mind will wander and "chatter," but the trick is sticking with the practice long enough to relax and improve concentration. Meditation reduces tension and helps relieve pain.

### Relaxation Techniques

A variety of methods produce the relaxation response. Deep breathing exercises have the potential to calm the sympathetic nervous system, reduce blood pressure, and decrease pain. Many people do not know how to breathe deeply from the abdomen, but once learned, this type of breathing is a tool available at any time to help produce a relaxed state.

During relaxation exercises, deep breathing is done from the abdomen and chest in a reclining or flat body position. Place your hand over your abdomen as it rises while you inhale for a count of three; you will feel the abdomen "deflate" as you exhale over a count of three. You will notice changes in your body after only a few cycles, but I recommend starting with ten slow deep breaths. If you breathe too rapidly, you may become dizzy, so keep your breathing slow. Use this simple breathing exercise along with other relaxation techniques to decrease the intensity of pain.

Progressive muscle relaxation is a technique that contracts muscles and then relaxes them, starting with the feet and moving up through your legs, hips, buttocks, torso, arms, hands, chest, neck, and up to the muscles in the face. Many bookstores and natural food markets have a selection of audiotapes with instructions for a step-by-step "trip" through the body. Progressive relaxation exercises should be performed gently, with minimal contraction in muscles that are the source of discomfort.

Be aware of the amount of tension generated as you contract the muscles and remember that muscles that have not been exercised may cramp when you first begin practicing this technique. This type of exercise is a good way to acquaint yourself with your body—we tend to forget about all the muscles we need for normal movement. The last step is tensing and releasing all your muscles at once. Always end a session with deep cleansing breaths, which increase the level of relaxation.

Relaxation techniques are free of side effects; just be careful not to stand up too fast and become dizzy and risk a fall. These exercises involve minimal or no expense, but you must put in the effort to gain the benefit.

## BODY SELF-AWARENESS

These techniques increase self-awareness of motions that increase pain and instability. Through improvement in movement, pain is decreased.

### Alexander Technique

F. Mathias Alexander was an Australian actor whose voice was chronically hoarse whenever he went on stage. Ineffective medical therapies frustrated him, and he embarked on his own search for help. Alexander discovered that the misuse of the neuromuscular activity of his head, neck, and spine caused the vocal dysfunction. He corrected these problems by recognizing the tensions and inefficient use of his body, and eventually he taught his techniques to others.

In essence, the Alexander technique is a mind/body movement reeducation course that heightens self-awareness of body movement and posture. The series of lessons demonstrates efficient ways to use painful joints and muscles so that movement takes less effort.

The Alexander technique is taught one-on-one in private lessons in which the teacher offers immediate feedback on harmful ways of holding and moving your body. A certified Alexander technique teacher is a highly trained professional who has completed sixteen hundred hours of training over a three-year period. Through the use of touch and words, the teacher coaches you to improve your standing, sitting, walking, bending, reaching, carrying, and lying down. Learning how to achieve balance with your own body goes along with an overall positive outlook. A course of therapy is about thirty private sessions, completed over fifteen weeks.

### Feldenkrais Method

Moshe Feldenkrais, an engineer and martial arts expert, developed an awareness of movement as a method to overcome a knee injury. This method involves education about movements and stretches that make you more aware of your posture as you bend, sit, stand, or walk. The method retrains your muscles to avoid positions that cause pain. Group lessons go through a series of small movements to increase range of motion and flexibility. Individual sessions involve moving through ranges of motion that allow greater awareness of body flexibility. A set of lessons usually includes two sessions a week for six weeks.

## MAGNET THERAPY

Many people, including some of my patients and some well-known sports figures, report remarkable relief of pain with magnet therapy, sometimes with the first use. Magnets are said to decrease muscle and joint pain, including back pain. They come in all shapes and sizes and are worn over the painful area. Magnets are placed in shoes, worn as necklaces, or are placed on beds like sheets.

However, we still don't understand how magnets are beneficial. We do know that static magnets do not make an electrical current unless they are passed though a coil of wire. Therefore, a stationary magnet on the skin would not be expected to generate a current. The mechanism that may play a role is the microcirculation in the blood vessels of the skin; this may generate the movement that results in an electrical current.

Numerous mechanisms have been suggested to explain why magnets work, including

- Improved blood and lymph circulation
- Interference with superficial pain nerve fibers
- Stimulation of acupuncture points
- Increased production of endorphins, the body's natural pain relievers

To date, no scientific research has proved any of these mechanisms, and some studies show mixed results. Nevertheless, additional studies are under way.

The possible side effects associated with long-term magnet use have not been determined, but if magnets are effective by producing local electrical currents, they may be toxic if left in place for extended periods of time. For example, if magnets increase blood flow, they should not be used with acute injuries since increased blood flow will exacerbate swelling. If you have a pacemaker, don't use magnets, because they can cause irregular heartbeats.

Static magnets probably have the best chance of working on abnormalities and decreasing pain on the surface of the body, such as superficial muscle spasm. The deeper the abnormality, the less magnetic force will help. Currently, magnets appear to have little toxicity, so they are assumed to be safe. I recommend using only magnets that are marked with their strength and manufacturer. If your pain is not better after a few weeks or so, try another remedy.

### Magnetic Melanie

Only one of my patients told me of positive results with magnet therapy. Melanie, age fifty-two, developed right-leg sciatica secondary to a herniated disc, and since she did not respond to medical therapy, she underwent a **discectomy**. Her leg pain improved, but her low back pain and stiffness came back about four months after surgery and her thigh pain returned. Melanie improved with NSAID therapy and a muscle relaxant, and she had physical therapy for range of motion exercises. Within two months she had decreased pain and improved motion, and although initially she was reluctant to tell me why she was better, Melanie finally told me that she thought her magnets had done the trick. A friend had told her about magnets, and she had decided to get a corset with magnets in place. At first, there was no response, but within a few weeks her back was less painful and she was able to do her exercises. She could not be sure, but she thought her magnets had made the difference. I was not ready to disagree with her, and since there was no overt toxicity, I told her to continue with her magnets. Although her back pain has improved, she continues to wear her magnets.

My magnetic patient may have seen benefits from the therapy because the source of her pain was localized to superficial layers of the back. Deeper structures may not be reached by the magnetic forces generated by static magnets. These abnormalities (osteoarthritis of the lumbar spine) may be more resistant to magnet therapy.

### Bracelets

Copper bracelets have been a complementary therapy for arthritis for many years. Whether copper deficiency causes arthritis has not been proven. The amount of copper needed each day is not known. I tell my patients that if their skin under the copper ornament is not green they are not absorbing any copper in any case. They are just wearing jewelry. Copper has to be in direct contact with the skin to be oxidized to be transported through the skin.

Bracelets of other metals have also been promoted as pain relieving. In some cases, the bracelets have been treated to be "ionized" to be more effective than nonionized bracelets. Experiments to demonstrate the benefits of one over the other have not been able to show a difference. What seems to be important for the wearers of bracelets is their belief that the bracelet will help their condition. Therefore, if you believe that your bracelet helps you, it will, whether it is "ionized" or not.

## HOMEOPATHY

Homeopathic remedies, developed at the end of the eighteenth century by Samuel Christian Hahnemann, a German doctor, are among the most frequently prescribed complementary therapies. One principle of homeopathy is "like cures like," meaning that a particular pattern of complaints can be cured by a drug that produces the same pattern of complaints in a healthy person. Another principle is that very small amounts of this drug have therapeutic value. The smaller the amount given, the greater the body's response. Some homeopathic drugs may be diluted to the degree that not even a single molecule of the original drug remains. In general, homeopathic remedies are believed to stimulate the body's ability to heal itself.

Homeopathic remedies may be tablets, liquids, or creams available from health food stores or pharmacies. These preparations contain so little medicine that most people can safely take them. You have little to lose when you try a homeopathic remedy if other therapies are not improving your back condition. But do tell your physician about these remedies. This advice is particularly important if your homeopathic practitioner recommends that you stop taking other medications. This could adversely affect your general medical condition, and remember that some medications should not be stopped abruptly.

## NUTRITIONAL SUPPLEMENTS

An overwhelming number of nonprescription supplements line the shelves of health food stores and pharmacies. Many are made from plants and herbs that were remedies before pharmaceutical companies were able to create the modern array of drugs. Aspirin is an example of an enduring plant-based remedy made from willow tree bark, which was known to decrease fever, headache, and muscle pain. It served as a plant-based therapy long before its active chemical, salicin, was identified by German pharmacologists.

Manufactured drugs are produced under supervision of governmental agencies and are subjected to quality-control testing so you have assurance about their purity and dosage measurement. Dietary supplements are not regulated by the Food and Drug Administration, and an article from the *Washington Post* reported that a 1998 California investigation discovered that about one-third of imported Asian herbals contained lead, arsenic, or mercury, or were spiked with drugs not listed on the label. In addition, without regulation, we don't know what part of the plant has the active ingredient, when it was harvested, or the storage conditions under which it was stored—all of which affect the potency. These issues have a direct effect on the usefulness of supplements you buy.

It's important to understand that not all "natural" plant therapies promote health—some plants are deadly. In books listing poisons, plants make up a significant number of agents that can stop the heart, cause low blood pressure, trigger convulsions, or result in coma. Never assume that "natural" is synonymous with "safe" or even "effective." Stick with plant remedies that have been subjected to research and testing.

Some dietary supplements offer complementary therapies to conventional interventions for acute and chronic low back pain. I always ask my patients to tell me if they are taking these supplements, because toxicities may occur in addition to or in spite of what the label on the bottle outlines. Don't start guessing about the possible cause of a new symptom when it could be related to a nutritional supplement.

Monitor your response in order to measure how you're doing. Has the pain decreased? Are you more functional? If the answers are yes, then increase your exercises and try to use less of your supplements over time. If the answers are no, then stop using the supplements and try something else.

The number of herbal supplements and their manufacturers continues to grow, which makes the choice of a single product difficult. Below are some guidelines that may be helpful:

- Choose a single supplement rather than a combination product; single agents have been studied, but the effects of combination products are more difficult to determine.
- Choose extracts over powdered preparations.
- Look for the FDA label describing the name and amount of supplement in the container.
- Choose products made by pharmaceutical manufacturers who are experienced in production of over-the-counter medications.
- Avoid products that describe miracle cures.
- Always take the supplement as described on the product label; if recommended doses are lacking or vague, don't take it.

### Devil's Claw (Harpagophytum procumbens)

Harpagoside, the active ingredient of devil's claw, comes from the plant root. The plant is an appetite stimulant and mild analgesic; low back pain studies using this herbal remedy were conducted in Germany. In one study, 118 patients with low back pain were treated with 50 mg per day of harpagophytum extract. A greater number of patients receiving active extract were pain-free when compared to the placebo group. In another study of 197 low back patients, a 100 mg dose of harpagophytum extract was found to be better than a 50 mg dose and placebo. Side effects included gastrointestinal symptoms, and the supplement is known to increase stomach acid secretion. Don't use it if you have a tendency to develop ulcers.

### Ginger (Zingiber officinale)

Ginger is one of the herbs used in Ayurvedic medicine, the traditional medical system and philosophy of India. This spice has properties that inhibit PG production. By decreasing PGs, ginger has potential as an effective anti-inflammatory and analgesic substance. Studies of osteoarthritis and muscle pain have shown that ginger supplements are effective in decreasing pain. The therapy had no side effects and remained effective for up to thirty months. Ginger and other Ayurvedic herbs (turmeric, frankincense, ashwagandha) take a month or longer to have an effect. However, once established, the beneficial effect may last for an extended period measured in months to years, without increasing the dose.

If you take ginger or any of these herbs regularly, be sure to tell your doctor, because these herbs in large doses can interact with prescription medications. For example, ginger can increase the effect of blood pressure and blood thinning medications, thereby causing low blood pressure and bleeding.

### Limbrel (Flavocoxid)

Limbrel is a medical food that inhibits the cyclooxygenase (COX) and lipoxygenase (LOX) enzymes. COX and LOX are enzymes that promote inflammation in the body. Limbrel is approved by the FDA for dietary management of the metabolic processes involved with osteoarthritis. Limbrel is not approved for the treatment of pain with osteoarthritis. However, individuals with difficulty taking NSAIDs because of stomach upset find benefits with taking Limbrel 500 mg twice a day without side effects. This food does not work rapidly. Some individuals need to wait weeks before they experience the full benefits of this agent. Limbrel is not a dietary supplement and is not intended for normal, healthy people. Limbrel is only available by prescription.

### Glucosamine and Chondroitin

These two supplements are promoted as treatments for osteoarthritis. Glucosamine sulfate, an aminosugar, which is a component of cartilage, has been available by prescription in Europe for years. Glucosamine comes from chitin, a substance extracted from the shells of crab, lobster, and shrimp. The usual allergy to shellfish is related to fish proteins, not the shells, so you should not be allergic to glucosamine even if you are sensitive to crab or shrimp. That said, a few of my patients have described sensitivity to glucosamine similar to what they experience with shellfish.

A Belgian study presented at the 1999 American College of Rheumatology meeting described glucosamine at a dose of 1500 mg per day as valuable in maintaining knee cartilage over a three-year period when compared to a placebo. However, problems with the X ray results have been raised, even though this study has been offered as positive data about the benefit of glucosamine for knee joints. No determination was made in this study about the effect of glucosamine on the lumbar spine. Cartilage in the knee is different from that in the lumbar spine end plates and discs, and glucosamine may not help disc disease. This point was made clear to me by one of my patients, with low back and knee pain.

Beth, seventy, had osteoarthritis of the knees and lumbar spine and had experienced symptoms for a number of years. I had treated her with a COX-2 inhibitor, which relieved pain symptoms in her knee and back. Prior to seeing me, Beth had been taking glucosamine sulfate for a number of months. Her knee pain improved but her back pain did not. Other patients have reported similar results.

I do not believe that glucosamine has a beneficial effect on back pain, but potential benefits for other joints currently are being studied. In addition, we do not have studies that report benefits or safety of glucosamine for more than a three-year time frame.

Chondroitin sulfate is a larger molecule than glucosamine and it may not be easily absorbed through the intestine and, thus, may not reach cartilage in joints. Cattle windpipes serve as the source of chondroitin used in supplements, because when derived from shark cartilage it may be contaminated with heavy metals such as mercury.

Chondroitin is taken 400 mg twice a day, but you may not see improvement for two months. Studies on chondroitin are fewer than those for glucosamine and any added benefit of chondroitin to glucosamine remains to be determined.

Chondroitin bears chemical similarity to heparin, a blood-thinning drug, so too many supplements may cause bleeding. If you bruise easily, or notice excessive bleeding when brushing your teeth, see your physician.

### SAMe (S-adenosylmethionine)

Available in Europe since the 1970s, SAMe has been used to treat both arthritis and depression. It is a biochemical formed in the body from the essential amino acid methionine (found in proteins) and adenosine triphosphate, a major energy source in the body. The interaction of the two helps form cartilage.

Studies have reported improvement in depression and arthritis. It appears that SAMe decreases pain in osteoarthritis of the hands and may increase finger joint cartilage. In a study of thirty-six patients with osteoarthritis of the knee, hip, or spine, 1200 mg of SAMe per day or 1200 mg per day of ibuprofen, taken for four weeks, were equally effective in decreasing pain, and both had similar side effects.

We still do not have good data about the role of SAMe in the treatment of acute low back pain, or the long-term benefits and toxicities of SAMe. The downside of SAMe therapy is that it is a dietary supplement without FDA supervision. In addition, a breakdown product of SAMe is homocysteine, associated with cardiac health risks.

### MSM: Methylsulfonylmethane

MSM is a derivative of dimethyl sulfoxide (DMSO), the chemical used to protect human tissues when they are frozen. It is also used in its medical-grade form to treat a bladder condition, interstitial cystitis. DMSO is a solvent passing molecules across membranes such as the skin and has been reported to cause fogging of the lens in the eyes of laboratory animals given the compound over extended periods of time. It also leaves a bad taste in the mouth and gives off a garlic aroma.

MSM has none of the bad characteristics of DMSO, including the garlic aroma. MSM does not require a prescription like DMSO does, since MSM is a dietary supplement. To date, no specific studies for MSM in low back pain have been conducted. MSM may take up to a month to work, and it appears that MSM isn't particularly helpful for acute low back pain. On the other hand, MSM may be beneficial as a complementary therapy for people with chronic low back pain. MSM comes as a 500 mg capsule. The recommended maximum dose per day should be found on the pill container. The side effects associated with a higher dose include diarrhea and cramps. If no effect is seen by the end of the second month on MSM, stop using it.

## DR. B'S PRESCRIPTION SUMMARY

- Complementary therapy should not replace conventional therapy.
- Tell your doctor about any complementary therapies, because they may conflict with or have an adverse effect on conventional treatment.
- Manual therapies such as chiropractic manipulation or massage can sometimes help decrease muscle pain. They are most helpful for age groups between twenty and fifty years of age.
- Mind-body therapies can help decrease stress through relaxation.
- Cognitive-behavioral programs are available on the Internet to help learn coping skills to relieve pain. This form of therapy can be one of the most effective and durable forms of complementary therapies.
- Acupuncture is now more widely accepted by conventional medicine as a way to offer additional pain relief.

# Chapter 12

# What to Know Before You Consider Surgery

SPINE SURGERY ALWAYS IS a trauma to your back. Even minimally invasive surgeries damage your skin, muscles, blood vessels, and discs. Healing takes time. In addition, surgery means that you no longer have all the pieces of your spine that you were born with, a situation that puts added pressure on the parts that remain. Alterations in spinal anatomy from surgery may be minimal or they may significantly modify the function of your spine. And the results of surgical intervention do not end when you are wheeled into the recovery room. For the rest of your life, the effects of surgery can unfold.

The United States has the highest number of spinal surgeries per capita in the world. European countries such as Sweden have fewer. Swedish surgeons are paid a salary independent of the number of the surgeries they perform, whereas in the United States many spinal surgeons are paid for each operation. This payment system encourages surgeons to consider operative solutions at an earlier point in the course of recovery. Some regions of the United States have higher rates of back surgery than others. The existing bias toward surgery may be related to experience of local surgical training programs toward earlier surgical intervention. However, a decrease in insurance preauthorization approvals and lowered reimbursement levels is reversing this trend.

## UNDERSTANDING THE RISKS

Every year hundreds of thousands of men and women undergo lumbar spine surgery because of low back and leg pain. The vast majority of these surgeries are appropriate and for most people the surgical outcome is excellent, but unfortunately we cannot say that surgery is successful 100 percent of the time.

A small but significant percentage of spine surgery patients have outcomes that are less than ideal, including

- Wrong operation for the spinal disorder
- Wrong surgical site
- Inadequate surgical correction
- Inexperienced surgeon
- Postoperative complications
- Anesthetic death

Most people do not think about these things when they choose surgery, although they do have some degree of fear. Surgeons are obligated to get your "informed consent" before they operate, and so they must describe the benefits and risks of each procedure. However, most people are focused on relieving their pain, and the human tendency is to think that bad outcomes happen to other people. Think again.

**When Surgery Is the Wrong Choice**

The days of exploratory back surgery are over. Now that we have new radiographic techniques, almost all back anatomy can be visualized without invading the body. A decision to undergo surgery should never arise from a sense of desperation. Consider all the facts first. For example, if your disc herniation is on the opposite side of your leg pain, then it is not the cause of your sciatica. Removing that disc will not help your pain. Remember our guideline: lumbar disc surgery is for leg pain, not back pain.

Surgery is questionable when pain or weakness has been present for months or years. A loss of function for years is not an indication for surgery because an operation does not lead to improved function. A surgical research project took a group of patients with stable neurologic deficits and operated on half of them. After three years, the nerve damage was similar in both the nonsurgical and surgical groups. In a stable situation, surgery is performed to achieve pain relief, not to improve function.

Do not have an operation just because you were injured at work and other employees have had a similar procedure. What worked for others may not apply to your situation, and an operation can seriously delay your return to work. In addition, be certain that the procedure is in your best interests and not those of your employer or physician.

### Is Surgery Right for You?

Surgery is indicated only if the clinical findings of leg pain correlate with physical findings and radiographic abnormalities. The specific cause of sciatica must be identified, and possible systemic disorders must be eliminated as potential causes of your back pain. In addition, MRI or CT findings must identify the correct anatomic level of disc herniation. Finally, you must understand the procedure and believe the benefits outweigh the risks. If all these factors coincide, surgery has an excellent chance of being successful.

Once you make the decision to undergo surgery, you must choose the best procedure to achieve the best results with the least risk for a bad result or complications. These days, a number of new technologies such as laparoscopes and lasers are used for spinal procedures. While these technologies are amazing, they are new, and accumulated experience is naturally more limited when compared to the more tried-and-true spinal surgical techniques. If you consider a new technique, be sure your surgeon has had extensive training and experience using it. In addition, you should know if the procedure is experimental or is actually an old technology being used in a new way. Of course, find out why the new technique is better than older, time-tested procedures for your particular situation.

### The Biblical Scholar

Father Mark, a fifty-six-year-old priest and biblical scholar, was having difficulty completing a book he was writing. At first he had difficulty with using his arms while sitting at his computer, and even lifting them to waist level caused severe pain. Naturally he was concerned that he would no longer be able to type. His first diagnosis was bilateral tennis elbows, and elbow bands and arm strengthening exercises allowed him to return to his computer to finish the first volume of his book.

The problem with his back started when he began the second volume, which put him in front of his computer for longer periods. Eventually he noticed increasing back and leg pain, which, at the beginning, was only in one side of his back. Standing up improved his pain, but his work demanded more time at the computer, which increased pain and progressively involved his buttock, his calf, and his foot. Eventually he was writing less and standing more. NSAIDs helped decrease pain, but his gastrointestinal tract did not tolerate these medications. An MRI scan revealed a herniated disc compressing the sciatic nerve, resulting in back and leg pain. Epidural corticosteroid injections were helpful but not curative, so after great soul searching, Mark decided to undergo a discectomy (partial removal of the herniated disc) and a foraminotomy (enlargement of the exit for the spinal nerve). The operation was a success, and he had almost immediate relief of his leg pain. Postsurgical back pain lasted about four weeks, and after six weeks he was back at his computer.

Our biblical scholar had a good result from his surgery and has continued to be pain-free, so for him, surgery was the right decision.

### Making the Decision

Keeping this background information in mind, you can begin to measure the risks and benefits of spinal surgery and determine if you are among the estimated 2 to 5 percent of people with back and leg pain who need surgery. In some circumstances, surgery can help those with sciatica feel better faster than medicines alone. For example, patients with nonoperative therapy for herniated discs have the same long-term outcomes (over a period of ten years) as those who have surgery, but the surgical group has more rapid relief of symptoms.

You may be a candidate for spinal surgery if you have

- Bowel or bladder incontinence (CEC syndrome).
- Progressive muscle weakness with a foot drop, or you are unable to walk on your heels or raise your toes—your weakness may reverse spontaneously, but the longer the weakness remains, the less likely it is that strength will return.
- Resistant, severe sciatica.
- Recurrent, incapacitating sciatica—you may have one sciatica attack that completely resolves, but soon after, pain down the leg returns and becomes increasingly severe; if the frequency and intensity of attacks interfere with your ability to work or enjoy typical activities of daily living, surgery is a worthwhile choice. In general, surgery is indicated when you experience a third recurrence of sciatica.

# DISCECTOMY

Open discectomy is the gold standard of spinal surgery and can initially bring good to excellent results in up to 95 percent of patients, provided they are appropriate candidates for the procedure. Minor complications occur in 4.7 percent of cases and the mortality rate is 0.03 percent.

This technique requires a three-inch incision in your back to expose the area of disc herniation and nerve compression and requires spinal or general anesthesia. Only the portion of the disc that is protruding and compressing the nerve is removed. The remainder of the disc is left in place to continue its work as a shock absorber. Extra bone may be excised (**laminectomy**) if the nerve is constricted in the spinal canal.

## Microdiscectomy

Microdiscectomy involves a one-inch incision, a high-magnification surgical microscope, and intense illumination. The advantages are improved visualization of the anatomy, less bleeding, and less trauma to the muscles in the spine. The success rate for microdiscectomy to relieve leg pain is 90 percent. The technique offers more rapid recovery time, earlier discharge from the hospital, and generally an earlier return to work.

However, this technique is not without concerns. Recurrence of disc herniation and tearing of the covering of the spinal canal (dura) occur more frequently with microdiscectomy. If the dura tears, the spinal fluid leaks out. This can cause headaches. Additionally, with a smaller incision, it is more likely the surgeon will not see pieces of disc or some nerve compression that has moved from the original location of the herniation. For this reason, a second operation often becomes necessary. Make sure your surgeon has extensive experience with microdiscectomy and firmly believes it will help you.

## Percutaneous Discectomy

Percutaneous discectomy is called the Band-Aid surgery. It is based on the premise that decompression of the nerve root can be achieved indirectly by entering the central portion of the disc and decreasing its volume, thereby resulting in the retraction of the disc herniation. Alternatively, if disc herniation is in an exposed position, not covered by vertebral bone, a probe placed through the skin during an X ray visualization can remove it. A tiny (one-centimeter) incision allows the entry of a surgical probe, and sedation and local anesthesia is all you need during the procedure. Once the procedure is completed, a Band-Aid covers the wound, thus the name.

Percutaneous suction discectomy removes the central disc material with a rotary blade and the pieces of the disc are vacuumed up through the probe. Some have reported a success rate as high as 85 percent, but others remain skeptical. Percutaneous procedures have been challenged by findings based on MRI studies that revealed no significant change in the appearance of the postsurgical herniated disc in the area of protrusion.

Percutaneous laser discectomy uses a laser at the end of the probe to vaporize the central portion of the disc. Laser energy is converted to heat in the disc tissues, which results in decreased volume of the gel in the disc. The procedure, which requires only local anesthesia, has reported improvement in about 75 percent of patients. The primary concern is achieving the appropriate amount of laser energy. Too much laser energy can damage surrounding tissues such as the nerve, vertebral endplates, or facet joints. This damage may then be a cause for chronic low back pain from a different source.

### Minimally Invasive versus Open Discectomy

At an international meeting of spine specialists, the relative benefits and risks of surgical discectomy were debated. Many of the points discussed at the debate have been described in this book. When the vote was taken, open discectomy was the choice of the experts. The most important aspect of surgery is adequate exposure of the abnormalities. Seeing the problem offers the best chance of success.

## SPINAL FUSION

It would be wonderful if we needed only superglue to get the bones to stick together. Unfortunately, a lumbar fusion is more complicated. The surface of the bone that is going to be fused is roughened so that a repair response is started. Then the surgeon places a new piece of your own bone, which is taken from your pelvic bone, to fuse over the roughened bone. Alternatively, allograft is used. This is bone taken from those who have left their bodies for medical science. Bone banks carefully screen bone donors for infectious illnesses, including AIDS and hepatitis. Using allograft means that a second incision in your body is not needed in order to have enough bone for a fusion. Sometimes the donor site for the fusion is more painful than the lumbar surgical site.

The basic idea behind a fusion is that your own bone cells will replace the graft bone over a six-to-twelve month period, during which time you will be in a spinal brace while the fusion "takes." The living fusion will become solid, offering stability to that segment of the spine. Sometimes the fusion may be augmented with metal hardware (see below) for added stability.

Fusion surgery is complicated and it doesn't always work. The non-union—where the fusion didn't take—may be a source of pain, independent of the original cause for the operation.

Current orthopedic research is looking at new ways to fuse bones. Certain bone proteins, when sprinkled on areas prepared for fusion, are able to get significant production of bone without the need for donor-site bone. When these are available, the success rate for fusion will increase.

Studies have demonstrated that one's overall health—not age—is the essential factor in deciding who is a candidate for spinal stenosis surgery. So, if you're in good general health, your age should not be an impediment to enjoying a better quality of life through surgery.

## SPINAL INSTRUMENTATION: THE HARDWARE STORE

The exhibit area at today's spinal surgery meetings looks like your neighborhood hardware store—one can wander around and examine a vast array of drills, hammers, screws, plates, and rods. This hardware can be placed in the spine with the intention of decreasing pain, improving function, and limiting instability. Spinal instrumentation is particularly important in people who have sustained significant trauma to the spine. Spinal rods can immediately stabilize fractures of the spine, and hardware can straighten scoliotic curves. On occasion, the bone grafted for fusion is stabilized with the addition of rods to decrease movement. Pedicle screws and cages, which are spacers between discs, are among the new hardware used to improve spinal conditions.

If you are considering surgery now, you need to know that your surgeon is familiar with the instrumentation used in your operation and that the hardware has been specifically designed for this problem and has a track record for reliability. Before the instrumentation is initially placed, you and your surgeon need to discuss the potential need to remove the hardware. You might assume that hardware in the body must cause pain, but that isn't the case. Once healing has occurred, the hardware causes no pain and you can function normally. Medical scientists are always developing new techniques and instrumentation to improve spinal care. Be sure you know the purpose of the procedure and the hardware, because it is always easier to leave hardware out than retrieve it later.

## The Five-Level Man

Juan, sixty, asked my advice about the deterioration of his back. His rheumatoid arthritis (RA) had been well controlled for over a decade, and the disease had not limited his activities. In fact, Juan still ran regularly, played tennis three times a week, and went hiking on vacations. However, while his RA was fine, his back was not, and he had developed increasing left thigh pain and numbness. NSAIDs, opioid analgesics, and epidural injections had diminished his pain but had not completely relieved it. Naturally he was frustrated because he was unable to do any of his recreational exercise.

X ray evaluation revealed multiple levels of severe disc degeneration from L1 to L2 and L4 to L5. An orthopedic surgeon evaluated Juan about his back pain and severe limited motion. After extensive discussions, a five-level laminectomy with fusion with five-level rod placement was completed. A postoperative infection was treated with antibiotics. After ten months he was walking four miles every day and was ready to start running on a treadmill. As an aside, his RA has remained under control and his arthritis regimen has not hindered recovery from his fusion operation.

About four years after his fusion operation, Juan had increasing pain in the back above the level of his fusion. His back had been fused, resulting in the loss of his lumbar curve, which placed stress on his upper spine. He underwent another procedure that removed his hardware and extended his fusion through the thoracic area. He returned to his physical activities once he healed but this took almost a year.

## THE ARTIFICIAL DISC—BUYER BEWARE

One of the most frequent questions patients ask me is "Is there a disc replacement?" Patients know that hip and knee replacements are successful operations. They assume that disc replacements must be available and as successful. Compared to other joint replacements that have been used for decades, the artificial disc has been available in the United States only since 2006.

The intervertebral disc acts as a universal joint in the spine. A universal joint moves front and back and side to side. The disc also acts as a spacer between the vertebrae. An artificial disc needs to move in all these directions to maintain the function of the spine. The artificial disc replacement has been engineered to maintain motion and reestablish normal relationships between the parts of the spine. The clinical implications of these relationships are that the disc can be the only abnormal portion of that section of the spine. The exclusions for a disc replacement include spinal joint arthritis, a herniated disc, scoliosis, osteoporosis, and spinal instability to name a few.

In addition, the surgical procedure is a more dangerous operation than the removal of a herniated disc. An artificial disc must be placed through an anterior approach to the spine. This approach requires the displacement of the major arteries, veins, and nerves that are situated in front of the spine. Damage to these vessels can result in significant blood loss. In addition, the disc replacement can be displaced or fracture the surrounding vertebrae.

Another concern involving disc replacements is the potential need to remove the disc if it fails. The number of failures has ranged from 7 percent to 45 percent in studied groups. Revision surgery is potentially dangerous because of the structures that need to be moved to remove the disc. Another question involves the best technique for replacement. Does a new artificial disc get placed (rarely) or is the space fused (usually)? These are issues that are actively investigated at this time. You should be aware of the whole story of artificial discs before you sign the consent.

## EMERGENCY SURGERY

Cauda equina compression syndrome (CEC) is a rare problem, but one that needs immediate spinal surgery. CEC causes bladder and bowel incontinence, loss of sensation between the legs (saddle anesthesia), and bilateral sciatica. This occurs when a large herniated disc compresses nerve roots at the end of the spinal canal, the cauda equina. CEC may also be caused by an infection in the epidural area or bleeding from blood-thinning medication. Pressure on the nerves causes the loss of neurologic functions, such as the ability to control the bladder and bowels. Control will not return unless pressure is taken off the nerve. Therefore, it's essential to remove the compression as quickly as possible.

CEC patients should receive immediate MRI evaluation of the spine to identify the cause and location of compression. They have little choice but to go forward with surgery to return neurologic function. The best results occur if surgery is performed within forty-eight hours. However, the decompression surgery should take place even if the compression has been present for days. Studies have demonstrated the slow return of neurological function with decompression surgery despite extended periods of CEC.

## ANTERIOR SPINE SURGERY

Most lumbar spine surgery is approached from the surface of the back, through the muscles, to the posterior portion of the vertebra. Operations that relieve compression of the nerves by the discs or joints can be carried out by this posterior approach. On occasion, an anterior approach through the abdomen to reach the front of the spine is necessary. Fusion of the lumbar spine can be accomplished in this manner. An anterior approach allows for the placement of bone between the vertebrae to form an interbody fusion. This approach may allow a greater opportunity for a successful result and improved mechanics of the spine but is associated with a greater number of possible complications. The intestines may be irritated by the procedure and may not work normally for days. Blood clots may occur more often in association with this approach. You should choose a surgeon with experience with this technique if you require this form of fusion operation.

## SPINE SPACERS

Patients with spinal stenosis develop symptoms of back and leg pain when they stand or bend backward. Extension of the spine narrows the space and causes compression of the nerves. If extension of the spine could be prevented, narrowing would be limited and compression prevented.

Prevention of extension of the spine is the idea behind the placement of spacers between the spinous processes of the lumbar spine. X-STOP is an interspinous process decompression system that elevates the vertebral bodies and limits extension. The X-STOP can also widen the corresponding neural foramen. The added benefit of the device is its percutaneous placement. That means the X-STOP does not require prolonged surgery for placement. The procedure may be done with local anesthetic and takes about an hour to complete. The benefits can be almost immediate. The device may be placed in individuals who are otherwise poor candidates for open procedures requiring general anesthesia because of serious medical problems such as renal or heart failure.

### The "Spaced" Grandmother

Grace is an eighty-year-old woman who was debilitated by her neurogenic claudication. She was concerned that she was going to be confined to her house because of her inability to walk. She liked playing with her grandchildren but was having increasing difficulties walking with them. She has general medical conditions that made surgical decompression a risky operation. She had two X-STOP devices placed. She is now able to walk with a cane for distances adequate for her to complete her daily tasks. She is pleased with her result since she is able to keep up with her grandchildren.

## CHOOSING AN ORTHOPEDIC SURGEON OR NEUROSURGEON

I've had the good fortune to work with excellent spine surgeons, and both orthopedists and neurosurgeons gain experience with these operations. Orthopedists with an interest in spine surgery usually take extra training to gain greater expertise with spinal procedures. Neurosurgeons may not learn about spinal instrumentation or fusion, but they have expertise in procedures that preserve spinal cord function. Either type of experienced spinal surgeon can perform the typical discectomy, laminectomy, or decompression operation. If a fusion or instrumentation is required, an orthopedic surgeon is usually part of the surgical team.

If you want the best chance for a good surgical outcome, then choose your spine surgeon carefully. This sounds logical, but the process may not be so obvious. As you know, surgery is subspecialized into different parts of the body. In order to gain experience, spine surgeons have extra years of training in the techniques used to fix fractures, straighten curves, remove pieces, and fuse them together. Here are some characteristics of good spine surgeons:

- Board-certified in a surgical specialty
- Recommended by your primary care physician or internist
- Recommended by a person you trust who had spine surgery
- Able to communicate with you about your surgery
- Extensively experienced with the procedure you require

Ask questions. You need confidence in your surgeon, and you should understand your procedure:

- How (and why) will it improve my condition?
- How long will it take to heal from my surgery?
- What are the potential surgical complications?
- Do my other medical conditions affect the success of the procedure?

You may not like the answers to these questions, but your surgeon should answer them before you have the surgery. If the surgeon doesn't want to speak with you before the procedure, it won't be any easier after the surgery. Always consider a second opinion, even if you are satisfied with your initial surgeon.

If your car needs bodywork you get two estimates before you would proceed. Surely your body is worth two "estimates." If both physicians agree on the need for surgery and the operative procedure, you can feel reassured. If they don't agree, at least you will be educated about differences of opinion. If you go to a neurosurgeon for the first opinion, try an orthopedic surgeon for the second. You can then decide which procedure makes the most sense to you.

### Preoperative Evaluation

Once you decide to have surgery, an evaluation is completed to determine your health status before the operation. You will have blood tests, including a test for clotting factors; an electrocardiogram; and depending on your age or smoking history, a chest X ray may be required. The older you are, the more tests you undergo. These evaluations identify potential problems that may occur during or after your operation.

Conditions such as diabetes, angina, high blood pressure, and so forth influence the way the anesthesiologist will treat you during surgery, and they affect your postoperative treatment as well. For example, you will stop taking baby aspirin to help prevent cardiovascular disease, and if you take an NSAID, you will stop one to four weeks before the surgery, depending on how long the drug stays in your body.

If you are taking a COX-2 inhibitor, you may not need to discontinue your medicine until the time of surgery. This is possible because the COX-2 inhibitor celecoxib does not interfere with the ability of platelets to stop bleeding.

Depending on the extent of the surgery, you may want to donate one or two units of blood; if a multilevel procedure is planned, two units are appropriate. Banking your blood decreases the risk of being exposed to infectious illnesses, even though they are rarely transmitted through blood transfusions.

If you smoke and have wanted to quit, now is a good time. Decreased lung function decreases oxygen to the tissues that are trying to heal. If you are having a fusion operation, smoking will increase the risk of nonunion. Smoking also increases the risk for lung infections. Some surgeons will insist on your quitting smoking before scheduling an elective fusion procedure.

Plan for your needs when you return home after surgery. If you live alone, prepare an area that will be comfortable and that has a clear path with no rugs on the floor between your chair and the bathroom. And speaking of the bathroom, renting a raised toilet seat can do wonders for making one of life's necessities a bit easier. In addition, try to prepare meals ahead of time and have them on hand in your freezer so you don't have to think about cooking.

## YOUR HOSPITAL STAY

Once you have had approval from your insurance carrier and the date has been set, you will enter the hospital. Unless you have multiple medical problems, you'll be seen the day of your operation. You will sign an informed consent form stating that you understand the benefits and risks of the procedure, but do not sign this form unless you are satisfied with the information you have received from your physician. Patients who have been fully informed and have chosen surgery have a better outcome.

The anesthesiologist will evaluate your medical history and allergies, if they are an issue. The anesthesiologist and surgeon will decide on spinal versus general anesthesia. During the procedure, you will receive an intravenous catheter to receive fluids and medications. If general anesthesia is used, medicine is given by vein to relax you while a tube is placed in your windpipe to control your breathing. If spinal anesthesia is used, a needle is placed in the spinal canal through which medication is delivered, and you will remain awake for the procedure.

After the surgery, you will be observed in the recovery room to be sure you are stable. Pain medicines for the postoperative period are initiated, first through a patient controlled analgesia (PCA) pump. The amount of medicine is controlled, but you can deliver it through the vein as you need it. Studies have demonstrated that when you have control over the timing of the pain medication, less is used than the amount you would receive when the medication is scheduled, and you obtain greater comfort.

You will be sent home from the hospital when you can eat and get out of bed. You will probably be stiff and have difficulty walking, but this is expected, particularly if you have had an open procedure.

## AFTER SURGERY—THE HARD PART

The most difficult part of the surgical process occurs after the operation when you reenter normal life. In the perioperative period, care must be taken with the surgical wound so that it heals without developing an infection. A nurse will generally discuss wound care before you are discharged from the hospital. Analgesic medications, some of which are opioid, are generally useful as you get used to doing daily activities for yourself.

To regain maximum function, you must move around. Initially, your body will try to keep all the cut tissues as still as possible to allow for healing. However, you must move these tissues to improve blood flow, which facilitates healing. At the beginning, movements are slow and small and repeated only a few at a time. As pain and time allow, you'll increase your movements.

Your goal is to obtain maximum motion with minimal pain.

### Physical Therapy

Physical therapy is part of your postoperative treatment. Physical therapists may seem to be mean taskmasters, but their expertise encourages you to improve your functioning in a sheltered environment. These health care professionals are trained to help you with normal activities, and they guide you in how long to sit or stand. Physical therapists can also help with comfortable positions to sleep at night. You also will learn how to get in and out of a car in the easiest way. In addition, physical therapists teach ways to perform various chores while limiting stress on the back. However, you should ask your doctor about performing more strenuous tasks such as mowing the lawn or vacuuming the carpets.

### Give Yourself Time to Heal

Although we would like to think in terms of weeks, healing within months is a more realistic goal. Getting better is hard work, and what once was done with very little energy seems like a major task now. I often tell patients to count to ten when they become frustrated by their limitations. This pause allows them to think about the way their back pain used to be. At least now they are on the road to recovery. In all likelihood, your recovery will take the same course as that taken by the vast majority of people who undergo successful back surgery.

## FAILED BACK SURGERY SYNDROME

Although spine physicians do not like to admit failure, they must acknowledge the group of patients who do not improve with their first back surgery. (Within all surgical groups, some patients do not improve.) If the pain was never improved, the initial surgery may have been done at the wrong level or the procedure may have been inadequate to reverse the abnormal anatomic changes. A second possibility is that another disc herniation has occurred at the same level. People in the latter group usually have a pain-free period before their leg pain returns. People with one herniated disc are at greater risk for another, and they may have a new disc herniation at a different spinal level.

Those with pain primarily in the back may have instability because the laminectomy may have been too extensive. Others develop a scar (epidural fibrosis) around the operative site surrounding the decompressed nerve. In addition to the development of a scar around the nerve, **arachnoiditis** may develop around the blood vessels surrounding the spinal nerves. Arachnoiditis can be associated with persistent chronic pain. Back and leg pain may occur six to twenty-four months after the initial operation.

### Epidural Fibrosis

Another operation may help correct these abnormalities. However, another surgical procedure will not alter the progression of arthritis or change the development of scar tissue. For this, you need nonsurgical management. Scar tissue (epidural fibrosis) removal through direct visualization remains experimental. In addition, the primary difficulty is not the removal of the scar but rather the means to control the inflammatory process so that no additional scar returns in the location where the original scar was removed. Gels and fat tissue are used to try to limit the development of epidural fibrosis and have had some success. The problem is identifying the individual who is at risk of developing scar. Those personal characteristics are not known. Epidural fibrosis remains a perplexing chronic disorder.

When you consider a second or third spinal operation, consult with a spinal surgeon who has experience with patients who have had multiple spinal surgeries. Physicians with this experience can make the difficult decisions about the potential benefits of another spine operation versus a nonoperative course. Everyone's usual tendency is to want to do something to make the situation better, and it takes mature experience to say no when others want to do a procedure even though it is more likely to harm than to help.

You may be a candidate for a spinal cord stimulator or an implantable opioid pump in the setting of severe, unremitting spinal pain after multiple surgical procedures. The stimulator consists of epidural electrodes that generate electrical signals that block pain transmission in the spinal cord. The electrodes are connected to a generator that is placed below the skin. The implantable opioid pump has a reservoir under the skin. A plastic tube is placed under the skin that travels to the spinal cord. Opioid medicine (usually morphine) is continuously directed to the spinal cord by a battery powered pump.

These therapies are limited to those individuals who have failed all other means to control pain.

## FUTURE SURGICAL TREATMENTS

Currently, researchers are investigating three new procedures for the treatment of disc degeneration. These invasive techniques have been helpful to people with back pain, but their long-term safety remains unproven.

Intradiscal electrothermal annuloplasty (IDET) is used for painful discs. An electrothermal catheter is threaded inside the disc. Released energy "cooks" the collagen in the disc like an egg, and the disc becomes stiff and loses its cushioning properties. However, patients are reported to have less back pain after this procedure. The exact mechanism that brings about the improvement is not yet clear. Only a small number of individuals have had this procedure, with only short-term follow-up. We need longer follow-up periods before we can confidently recommend this procedure.

Genetic therapies are in the experimental stage for restoring discs. Genes that produce collagen can be incorporated in the DNA of viruses. The genes are transferred to disc cells by the "altered" viruses. The disc cells then make increasing amounts of new disc components.

However, a number of questions surround gene therapy. Will the new gene products be used by disc cells to reform disc components? How long will these genes remain active? Will the procedures need to be repeated? Will these cells spread to other discs? To other parts of the body? A significant amount of research will be needed before gene transfer becomes an accepted surgical treatment for spine disorders.

Disc transplants remain experimental. Heart transplants and kidney transplants are successful because good blood flow can be established to the new organs to assure their survival. Discs are entirely different. Blood flow comes through the surrounding bone. That requires transplanting a single structure including the vertebral endplates and the disc to have a successful operation. A larger disc requires greater blood flow. Without blood flow, nutrition to the tissues is lost resulting in rapid degeneration. This is particularly a problem with lumbar discs that are larger than cervical ones. In the final analysis, a better result can be achieved with a fusion operation.

## DR. B'S PRESCRIPTION SUMMARY

- At least 5 percent of back patients require spine surgery.
- Over 90 percent of spine surgeries are successful.
- The first surgery for a herniated disc or spinal stenosis has the best chance of success.
- Remember, disc surgery is for leg pain, not back pain.
- When a back injury or degenerative condition causes loss of bowel or bladder function, leg weakness, or intolerable pain, immediate surgery is usually necessary.
- Before you agree to surgery, always ask questions about the short- and long-term side effects, and be sure your surgeon has extensive experience treating others like you.
- An intervertebral spinous process spacer is worth consideration if an open decompression operation is not possible.
- In general, open procedures versus minimally invasive procedures tend to have a better outcome.

Part III

# LIVING WITHOUT BACK PAIN

Chapter 13

# Lower Your Risk for Back Pain with Prevention

## *The ABC Plan*

THE CONCEPT OF PREVENTION does not have a great track record, and this dismal situation is true not only for back pain but for most health issues. It's really quite simple. Healthy people lack motivation to participate in preventive activities. They wait until they have their back attack (or other illness) and then try to prevent a recurrence.

Once you have had one back attack, you are at greater risk of having another within a year. Some studies suggest this is true for as many as 50 percent of back pain sufferers. However, the second attack is usually milder than the first. The second attack occurs because people forget the lessons learned from the first back pain episode. They go back to their old habits and lift objects from awkward positions, stretch too far, or sit too long.

Do not become a repeat back offender. Remember what caused your first back attack. Practice good body mechanics, rest when appropriate, and exercise at the correct time of the day (generally later in the day). If you follow these simple rules, a second attack of pain is less likely. Here are my guidelines for avoiding back problems—and preventing them from recurring.

If you remember your ABCs, you will go a long way in preventing back problems to begin with.

### A—ABSTAIN FROM SMOKING

If you are a smoker, make every effort to stop now—your back, along with your lungs and heart and other organs, will thank you. All the tissues of the body require oxygen to maintain their function, and smoking robs these tissues—especially your spinal discs—of the optimal amount of oxygen. Because no blood vessels supply the interior of the discs, all the oxygen has to seep in from the surface. If the blood contains less oxygen, the discs receive less, too, and lack of oxygen is part of the disc disintegration process that increases the risk of herniation. This also has implications for more rapid disc degeneration resulting in facet joint arthritis and spinal stenosis.

## B—BETTER BODY MECHANICS

The spine is a beautifully engineered structure, and we know posture is good if someone can effortlessly maintain normal position and movement for extended periods of time. Maintaining normal posture is a function of the ligaments that support the spine and legs and also of normal tension in muscles. When any component of the balanced spine is moved off center, this effortless state is altered (fig. 13.1).

Figure 13.1.    Good and poor posture. The left figure has good posture with the head over the pelvis with normal spinal curves. The right figure has poor posture with a flat low back. The flat back causes a forward bend of the knees and neck. This posture fatigues all the muscles of the neck, back, and legs.

Every day, your spine enables you to accomplish a number of tasks without pain. Think of it. Your spine supports your body when you lift a large object, and it stays straight when you make it sit in a car on a drive from Washington, D.C., to Boston, with only one stop for gasoline. If your spine is positioned correctly while you accomplish these tasks, you will suffer no ill effects. However, if a heavy load is off center, which twists your back, or if the car seat offers no support, you will probably develop back pain.

If I had to choose the one position that causes the most difficulty with back pain, I would point to a twisted or rotated spine. Back pain frequently occurs when lifting even minimal weight with a twisted posture. When the spine twists, it is at a mechanical disadvantage. The muscles are stretched on one side and short on the other, and, therefore, they are unable to generate the usual support force to the spine. The joints of the back are compressed unnaturally and the added pressure of lifting a weight only causes more damage to the structures.

Rachel, a twenty-two-year-old college student, moved into a fourth-floor apartment in a building without an elevator. She had driven a number of hours, and carrying the furniture up four flights of stairs took the rest of the day. The mattress was particularly difficult to maneuver, but instead of getting help or pushing the mattress while facing it, Rachel twisted her back to lift it onto the bed. Immediately the injured muscles started to tighten and her range of motion was limited the rest of the day, making the rest of the move very difficult. It took four weeks before the muscle tightness resolved.

Rachel's story highlights the risk associated with bad body mechanics and physical tasks. Think about the way you lift an object before you do it, instead of trying to figure out why your back is painful afterward.

**Lifting Posture**

When lifting any object, your feet and your back should be going in the same direction. You should face the object, bend your hips and knees, and lift with your legs, not your back. The object should be kept as close to your body as possible. If you can, it is better to lift the object from a height as opposed to lifting it from the ground.

If you must lift heavy objects frequently, consider using an abdominal corset to increase intra-abdominal pressure to support your spine. These corsets are not magic—they don't work if they aren't closed around your body. At one of the local hospitals, I noted that many of the hospital employees leave the corsets open. A recent study showed that most people who are given instructions about using abdominal corsets still use them incorrectly. However, the corsets may be helpful, even if left open, if it makes you remember to lift with your legs, not your back.

## Standing Posture

Standing in one position for a length of time can lead to fatigued muscles in your lower back. You may have experienced this feeling at a party where no chairs are available, or in a museum with no place to sit down. The upright posture increases the curve in the lumbar spine and stretches the muscle (psoas) in the front of the spine that travels to the hip. Lift one leg to rest on a stool. Transfer weight from foot to foot, or flatten your back with a pelvic tilt (see chapter 10). These positions take pressure off the psoas muscles and the curve of your back. Do these with any activity that requires prolonged standing, such as ironing, giving a lecture, or painting a wall.

## Sitting Posture

A good sitting posture requires that the height of the seat allows your feet to be flat on the floor, with your knees at slightly above 90 degrees. The back of the chair should support the lumbar curve. Chairs used in offices have an adjustable back and wheels, and the tension and position of the back support should be adjustable along with the height of the seat.

### Choosing a Chair

If you are experiencing back pain, the best chair for you has a firm upholstered seat, with a firm straight back and armrests. Wait to use the soft, sofa-type chair when your back pain has totally resolved. In a soft chair, your back is constantly making adjustments to support your spine, and these tiny adjustments can cause fatigue or increase pain because your back is working very hard. When you sit in a chair with firm support, the muscles can relax because the chair supports them.

## Stretching Posture

Many of us get into trouble when we stretch. You're the last one on the plane, so you have to stretch to squeeze your carry-on bag into the overhead bin between suitcases that seem to weigh a ton. Or you have to stretch across the bed to tuck a sheet under the corner. Maybe a bag of groceries has shifted to the farthest recesses of your car trunk. In these situations, you may stretch to reach, only to recognize that you are about a foot too short for the task! About five seconds later, the muscles in your low back and side have realized this fact, too, and now they are in spasm.

The simple answer to overstretching is to get closer to the object you want to move. If it is above your head, get a step stool. (If it's in an overhead airline bin, ask for help.) If you must reach the other corner of the bed, put one knee on the mattress and move closer to the corner. Instead of bending over to vacuum, kneel down on your knee to keep your back straight, depending on the type of vacuum you have, of course. Place packages in the front of the trunk, or on the backseat of the car.

## Avoid Back Fatigue

Never stay in one position for an extended period of time. Whether you're standing or sitting, change the position and move around at least once an hour, more frequently if your back quickly fatigues. Constant contraction of muscles makes them fatigue, and once that happens, they start to ache. Aching muscles are weaker muscles, and once their functioning is compromised, you are at greater risk for injury.

It's easy to forget simple prevention tips. For example, you may sit like a prisoner on an airplane. But take a stroll to the lavatory even if you don't need it. If you sit at a computer, remind yourself to get up to get your muscles moving. If you spend hours on the phone for your job, get a headset if possible, which allows you to get up and walk around. All these activities improve the function of your lumbar spine, and it will thank you by aching less.

## Maintain Fitness

When you are physically fit you are at less risk for developing low back pain. We can define fitness in a number of ways. For example, cardiovascular fitness is the ability to climb stairs or run without getting short of breath. In a study of firefighters, those in good physical condition had significantly decreased risk of back pain compared to those in poor physical condition.

Strong back muscles represent another type of fitness. Compared to other muscles in the body, the muscles in the back are generally weak;

if we increase strength in these muscles, we can decrease our risk of developing low back pain. While this is important for everyone, it is essential for those whose jobs require heavy lifting and physical labor. Exercises that strengthen the muscles in the front (abdominal flexors) and in the back (back extensors) can decrease your risk of injury if you lift heavy objects or twist and bend frequently while at work.

Do your general fitness exercises every other day. The day off allows your body to revitalize muscles fatigued by the exercise. Engage in an exercise program vigorous enough to stimulate about thirty minutes of perspiration. "Breaking a sweat" means you have used enough calories to generate heat, which is a sympathetic nervous system response that benefits the part of the nervous system that inhibits pain. These types of exercise also improve circulation, flexibility, and muscle tone.

## C—CORRECT DIET

Making wise choices about the foods you eat can be healthy for a number of reasons. Too many times my patients have promised me that they will be thoughtful about what they will eat. They make commitments that are hard to keep. At times they have very little information about nutrition to know what a correct choice is. A number of diets are available to control calories. Pick one that works and stick with it.

### Get Plenty of Antioxidants in Your Diet

Make sure your diet contains abundant amounts of fruits and vegetables, which are good sources of vitamins A, C, and E, the antioxidants. Beta-carotene is found in green and yellow fruits and vegetables like cantaloupe, apricots, spinach, and carrots. Dairy products and eggs provide vitamin A, citrus fruits are loaded with vitamin C, vegetable oils supply vitamin E.

Scientific evidence proving the direct benefit of antioxidants on intervertebral discs is still lacking. Although I do not have the clinical trials to prove it, I believe that antioxidant supplements have the potential to slow oxidative damage to the spine. Discs of the spine are one of the places that might benefit from this therapy. An adequate dose of antioxidants, preferably from food, is important to maintain spine health.

Our exposure to free radicals is part of the ongoing aging process throughout the body, including the spinal discs. In an autopsy study of people aged thirteen to eighty-six, oxidative damage was identified in cartilage cells in the middle of the discs. The damage started in the teenage years and continued in each age group. In addition, evidence of the body's attempts to repair the oxidative damage was present in all examined discs. This study confirmed the notion that disc degeneration from oxidative damage starts in the second decade of life.

These active oxygen molecules (free radicals) attach to cells in your spinal discs and cause damage. The cells try to repair the injuries but are ineffective, which means the disc wears out too soon. Antioxidants (vitamins A, C, E, and beta-carotene) are able to neutralize the damaging effects of oxygen radicals.

If you take these nutrients as supplements, keep in mind that the fat-soluble vitamins A and E are absorbed and stored with fat and thus are eliminated very slowly. Excessive amounts can accumulate in the body and become toxic. Health problems associated with taking these antioxidant supplements at levels above the recommended limits include kidney stones and diarrhea with vitamin C, increased bleeding in people taking anticoagulant medicines with vitamin E, and hair and nail breakage with selenium. Doses of vitamin A at a level of 100,000 units are toxic. The National Academy of Sciences has recently set "upper intake levels" for vitamins C and E and the mineral selenium as follows:

- Vitamin C: 2000 mg
- Vitamin E: 1100 mg (synthetic)
- Selenium: 400 mcg

### Vitamin D and Calcium

Remember that it is never too early to start thinking about calcium to make our bones strong. Up to age ten, 800 mg a day is a good recommendation. During adolescence 1500 mg is required during active growth. This also is an amount recommended during pregnancy. In mature adults, 1200 mg is adequate. Vitamin D has recommended levels that range from 400 international units (IU) to 2000 IU. Currently, the general consensus is that many individuals are vitamin D deficient. The higher level of 2000 IU will likely be the recommendation for those who have limited exposure to sunlight, gastrointestinal malabsorption, and nutritional deficiencies.

Moderation is the best policy. Get the vitamins you need from nutritious food. Do not go overboard. Too much of a good thing can cause harm.

### Maintain a Good Body Weight

Obesity in itself is not a risk factor for the development of low back pain, but it prevents you from doing exercises properly and comfortably. If obesity results in a sedentary lifestyle, then all the risks associated with inactivity remain present. For most people, the body mass index (BMI) has been a good measure for whether or not you are overweight. For example, if you are six feet tall and weigh 200 pounds, your BMI would be 27, which is a bit high. You would do better at a weight of 170 or 180. If you are five-foot-five and weigh 150 pounds, you would have a BMI of 25. Guidelines from the National Institutes of Health define overweight as a BMI greater than 25. Obesity starts at a BMI of 30.

Recently, questions have been raised about the BMI and whether this number is the ideal body weight for individuals. Experts have suggested that a healthy body weight might be slightly higher. The suggestion was that the presence of a modest amount of body fat was an indication of a healthy status. Also the presence of extra calories could help sustain an illness that would affect food intake.

These suggestions do not give you license to consume cheesecake every night to get to your "healthy" weight. Being at a weight that allows you to function without excessive fatigue, shortness of breath, or muscle aches is a weight you should try to maintain.

## KEEP WORKING

When back pain is related to your job, it is often complicated by the interaction with your employer and the workers' compensation system. And if you were unhappy with your work environment, that could prolong your back pain as well as your return to work. You need to be compensated fairly for loss of working time, and you also need to modify the conditions at your job that caused the back attack in the first place, whether you have a desk job or one that is physically strenuous. It's important to return to work, in any capacity, early in the course of a back attack. The longer you are out of work, the less likely it is that you will ever return to gainful employment. If someone is out of work for one year after a back injury, the chances of returning to a job are essentially zero. Max, a forty-five-year-old office worker, came to my office three days after the onset of pain associated with a lifting accident at his work. His office was moving to another location in the building, and he had been lifting boxes for two days. He developed pain and stiffness in his back that made it impossible for him to sit at his desk. He had muscle strain associated with lifting (he had twisted his back frequently). He was treated with medications and a five-day sick slip. When he returned to my office, his back pain had improved and his muscle spasm resolved. He was sent back to work with the recommendation that he be excused from any additional lifting associated with his office move. He was encouraged to move frequently during the day. With the modification in his work duties for three weeks, Max had total resolution of his back pain and has returned to his usual job.

The therapies in my basic back pain relief program can help you if you were injured at work. Once you are pain free for five to ten days, returning to work is feasible. Don't carry objects greater than ten pounds initially, even if your job involves heavy lifting. Always use good body mechanics—your feet and face are in line, with no spinal twisting. As you feel more comfortable with lighter lifting tasks, you can progress to lifting heavier objects. If you sit for most of the day, remember that sitting puts strain on the lumbar spine. Get up frequently to relieve back muscle fatigue.

---

### DR. B'S PRESCRIPTION SUMMARY

- Back pain can be prevented—the ABC Plan.
- A—Abstain from smoking now.
- B—Better body mechanics are important to maintain general physical fitness and comfortable posture.
- C—Correct diet includes antioxidants and other essential nutrients including calcium and vitamin D and healthy calories.
- Achieve and maintain an appropriate body weight.
- Go back to work once your pain resolves.
- Maintain the strength of your bones with exercise and supplements.

# Chapter 14

# Enjoying Sex without Hurting Your Back

"WHEN CAN I HAVE SEX AGAIN?" I wish I heard this question more often, but unfortunately, many men and women are reluctant to ask about sexuality. Perhaps you want to be intimate with your partner but you're worried that the act itself will make your condition worse. Your partner may feel the same way, and he or she may shy away from intimacy with you, with the kindest of intentions. Still, you may see it as rejection. These are the kinds of misunderstandings that can occur when back pain is an issue.

Ignorance and lack of communication lead to misconceptions about sexual health and low back pain. On the other hand, honest, caring discussions, along with psychological support, lead to a strong emotional and sexual bond despite the presence of low back pain. Obviously, the information presented here is not meant to serve as a manual covering all the issues related to sexual health, but rather, it concentrates on helping you remove the barriers that may have formed because of low back pain.

First, the outlook for people with acute low back pain is different from the outlook for chronic pain sufferers. Acute back pain is intense but will resolve, and a short hiatus from sexual activity is easier to tolerate when you expect the problem to resolve. But with chronic back pain you may need to modify sexual activity in order to have a successful relationship.

## IT'S NOT ALL PHYSICAL

When no health concerns exist, you and your partner are free to explore a variety of body positions during lovemaking. Spontaneous experimentation may have no consequences other than slight muscle soreness the following day. Under those circumstances, sexual climax may be the measure of a successful interaction. But, as we all know, a healthy sexual relationship involves more than physical lovemaking. Sexual intercourse is only a small part of a complex interaction of emotional and physical factors. We sustain partnerships by demonstrating our concern for the other person and by expressing our romantic and affectionate feelings in nonsexual ways, too.

You have a choice when it comes to sex. You can decide that modern society is too caught up with sex, and besides, thanks to media images, only a rare person can reach these ambitious sexual goals. So you conclude you're better off not worrying about your sexual needs while your back hurts. You can live without sex, so why bother?

Don't give up so fast. A healthy sex life can have beneficial effects on your back pain—and on your general health, too. Sex is a workout for your cardiovascular system, and you also burn a few calories. When you have sex, blood flow increases, which improves the appearance of your skin. Orgasm causes the release of endorphins, chemicals in the brain that act as the body's natural analgesics. Endorphins promote restful sleep and a general sense of well-being. So, indeed, sex is worth the trouble.

If you have acute low back pain, a short respite of a few days may allow your back pain and spasm to improve and sexual movements will not cause increased pain. If you think these sexual motions may increase your discomfort, practice them without your partner. If you don't notice increased discomfort, then sex with your partner is likely to go well. However, if pain occurs with simple movements of the back, wait a bit longer. If your pain is chronic, then you'll need to plan your sexual activity more carefully.

### Talk Is a Sexy Word

In 1998, in an article published in *Arthritis Today*, Jackson Rainer, Ph.D., said that his favorite four-letter word for intercourse is "talk." Dr. Rainer suggests that romantic interactions can occur when we're sitting together at the kitchen table fully clothed. Of course, the implication is that various levels of communication lay the groundwork for a caring, successful relationship. This is never more important than in the presence of physical limitations. You and your partner need to discuss your respective concerns and ask questions that will lead to greater understanding of the problem you're dealing with. For example:

- What makes your pain worse?
- What activities do not cause pain?
- When is the best time for intimacy?

In addition, both you and your partner may need reassurance about desirability. Do not wait until you are making love to talk about these issues, but instead, plan ahead in order to make the interaction painless and enjoyable. Don't forget romance! Nonphysical interactions support your relationship, and these can include a variety of things from compliments about your partner's appearance to appreciation for his or her emotional support to simple acts that show depth of feelings.

## PAINLESS POSITIONS

The best way to find comfortable positions during sex is to re-create the positions that are comfortable to your lower back during everyday activities. For example, if the back support of a particular chair is good, then use that chair for sexual intercourse. Or find the position in bed that causes the least discomfort for your spine. In order to decrease strain on your back, here are some general guidelines:

- Avoid positions that increase the low back curve—that motion causes pressure on the facet joints.
- Avoid lying flat on your stomach.
- Avoid bending forward at the hips with your legs straight—this causes stretching of the sciatic nerve and hamstring muscles.
- Keep the amount of weight your partner puts on your body to a minimum. Place your hands on the bed to support your weight.
- Avoid the man-on-top "missionary position." For men this position increases lumbar lordosis and stretch on low back muscles. For women on the bottom, any movement of the pelvis will require extension of the spine and increased pain.
- The partner without pain should supply the most motion.
- A flat lower back and upward lift to the pelvis (pelvic tilt) is pleasant and protective.

Figures 14.1 through 14.4 show positions that offer maximum comfort during sexual intercourse for men and women. The type of motion matters, too. Rapid thrusts may cause too much discomfort, whereas

Figure 14.1.    Spoon position.

Figure 14.2.    Straddle position.

Figure 14.3.    All-fours position.

Figure 14.4.    Rocking chair.

slow, gradual movements may be less painful and allow for a different sensation than the more athletic activity associated with unrestricted sex. My advice to partners is to tell each other what positions and touches are pleasant and stimulating and to develop signals between you that acknowledge the onset of pain with particular movements.

The spoon position (fig. 14.1) offers the greatest safety for both partners. Pillows strategically placed on the bed can offer correct support to the head, pelvis, and thighs. Both partners have their hips and knees flexed with a pelvic tilt. The flat back protects the facet joints, and the bent hips and knees take the tension off the sciatic nerve and the psoas muscles. Either partner can supply the pelvic movement that offers genital stimulation.

The straddle position (fig. 14.2) may be used with your partner looking toward you or away from you. The partner with back pain should determine the most comfortable position. This position allows your lover's weight to be placed on the bed or your knees (and not your back).

The all-fours position (fig. 14.3) allows sexual intercourse with the partner with back pain to support body weight with the arms. A flexed posture with slow thrusts is possible with this position. If a woman has back pain in this position, it may be best to have a more sturdy foundation on the floor, instead of a bed. With both partners' knees on the floor and a support under the woman's torso, movement of the pelvis will not "rock the boat" and cause involuntary, painful muscle contractions. Speaking of rocking, a rocking chair without arms may offer back support as well as pelvic motion (fig. 14.4). Variations on these themes are allowed as pain decreases.

When low back pain is present, not all sexual difficulties are related to the discomfort itself. Fortunately, erectile dysfunction is rarely related to abnormalities in the lumbar spine, but sometimes the therapies for low back pain may contribute to poor performance. For example, antidepressant medications used for chronic pain as well as depression can cause sexual dysfunction with inhibited ejaculation in men and decreased orgasm in women. Antidepressants can also cause vaginal dryness that results in pain during intercourse. Opioid medications can decrease pain but also may blunt sexual desire or response, and muscle relaxants may have a similar effect. In addition, excessive alcohol intake is known to suppress libido. Our challenge with medication is to find a balance between a large enough dosage to control pain, and a dose low enough to limit toxicity, including sexual impairment.

Fatigue interferes with successful sexual performance, and fatigue only amplifies pain. The old adage "plan ahead" certainly applies to eliminating fatigue. If you desire a successful sexual encounter, then make sure you're well rested.

### Sexual Satisfaction at Sixty

Tom, age sixty, had low back pain from osteoarthritis of the spine. After six months of treatment, his pain had improved but not enough for him to continue a satisfactory sexual relationship with his wife. The missionary position was particularly bothersome. He had been doing flexion exercises earlier in his treatment, but he had stopped them a few months before I saw him. He was taking ketoprofen in a sustained-release form for his pain. I suggested an additional dose of ketoprofen or acetaminophen prior to sexual activity, and I suggested alternative sexual positions. This combination proved successful, and eighteen months after my recommendations, his low back pain was improving and his sexual function is better as well.

Tom's case illustrates that sexual performance can benefit from careful timing of medication. To allow for adequate analgesia, take your pain medication two to four hours before planned sexual activity.

If sexual climax cannot be achieved through intercourse, then you and your partner should discuss alternative techniques. This may be difficult if there are social, cultural, or spiritual barriers to oral sexual stimulation, but I recommend discussing these issues because situations exist in which back pain limits the ability to engage in sexual intercourse. In addition, those with increased tension in sex organs that prevents orgasm through other means should consider self-stimulation. Releasing sexual tension by any of these means decreases muscle contraction and increases endorphin levels.

## SEXERCISES

Exercise helps improve sexual satisfaction, and any form of aerobic exercise improves cardiovascular function and increases stamina. In particular, Kegel exercises for the pelvis increase sexual enjoyment for women by strengthening the pelvic floor muscles supporting the bladder, uterus, rectum, and vagina. These are the muscles that contract around the penis during intercourse. Kegel exercises may also have some benefit for men. Improvement may be possible for premature ejaculation and erectile dysfunction. Improved strength of the pelvic floor may enhance control of sexual response and enhance pleasure.

Kegel exercises are easily performed while urinating. Slowly contract the pelvic floor muscles, a motion that halts urine flow. Hold the contraction for ten seconds, release, and repeat the contraction several times. The same muscles can be contracted at other times while standing, sitting, or lying down. Do twenty-five to fifty contractions twice a day.

## BACK SURGERY AND SEXUAL FUNCTION

Fusion of the lumbar spine can be accomplished by a posterior or anterior approach. A posterior approach avoids the autonomic nerves placed in the anterior portion of the lumbar spine. An anterior approach has a greater probability of dislodging these nerves. These nerves are involved with sexual arousal, male ejaculation, and female orgasm. Studies have reported the benefits of fusion surgery on reduction of pain. As a result of pain reduction, sexual quality of life improved. However, the benefits were not equal in the surgical groups. Posterior fusions had four times less difficulties with sensory problems or disturbed ejaculation compared to those who underwent anterior fusions. About 20 percent of women who underwent either form of fusion reported a decrease in genital sensation and disturbed orgasm. These reports suggest that men should consider a posterior fusion if they want to minimize the risk to sexual function. About one in five women will experience a decrease in sexual function with either procedure.

## Additional Consultation

If you continue to have sexual difficulties beyond that of back pain alone, consider seeking help from a sex therapist or a psychiatrist. Back pain is sometimes used as an excuse for limiting sexual relationships. Or, if your relationship is already troubled, then back pain may further complicate your problems. Simply changing your sexual position is not enough to change feelings, and a solution can be found only through improved communication. Consider additional help if necessary, but do not let your relationship deteriorate.

A healthy and understanding sexual relationship is a part of the complete prescription for a better back. You do not have to forgo the pleasures of this human interaction just because you have back pain. Intimacy goes beyond the act of sexual intercourse. When pain hinders your relationship, other means of sexual arousal can be used to broaden the ways of satisfying the needs of your partner. The benefits are worth the effort.

---

### DR. B'S PRESCRIPTION SUMMARY

- Back pain should never prevent you from having a successful sexual relationship.
- Sexual intimacy has multiple health benefits.
- "Talk" is a sexy four-letter word.
- Practice the most painless sexual positions, such as keeping your back flat, and avoiding the missionary position, which increases the curve to your lower back.
- Talk with your doctor about your medications if you think they are limiting your sexual performance.
- Lumbar fusion may help sexual function when a posterior approach is used.

# Epilogue

## *Being Back in Control Will Heal Your Back!*

YOU SHOULD NOW HAVE A GOOD IDEA how to put together the parts of your prescription that will work for you. I have mentioned a wide range of therapies that are effective for low back pain. I prefer active therapies to passive ones. That is my bias. Active therapies leave you in charge so you can control your recovery—back in control. That is also why I prefer conventional therapies over complementary. Many complementary therapies, in addition to being time-consuming, require the intervention of others.

Currently, research signals great hope for major advances in prevention, diagnosis, and treatment of back pain. Genetics research will help us understand hereditary factors that predispose to the development of disc degeneration. We will identify environmental factors that cause disc degeneration so we can prevent it. More sensitive diagnostic tests will allow us to visualize the spine in motion and see injured muscles clearly. More effective and less toxic NSAIDs are possible. Nonopioid forms of pain therapy are in development. Artificial disc replacements are being tested, and new fusion techniques won't require taking bone from the pelvis. The increasing interest in occupational therapy is shedding new light on ergonomic factors that limit the risk for back pain at the workplace. The future will improve our understanding of the factors that cause back pain. Our ability to take care of the persons with back pain will also improve.

Until that time, educate yourself about your back. Being educated will promote your improvement and save you exposure to diagnostic tests or therapeutic interventions that can have more risks than benefits. Use your knowledge with your primary care physician, with your physical therapist, with your anesthesiologist, with your massage therapist. Ask questions. Be critical of the answers. Decide what makes the most sense to you. Being in control will Heal Your Back.

- Be active in your recovery.
- Be informed.
- Keep moving.
- Use medicines as needed.
- Do exercises to remain strong.

# Glossary

**acupunture.** The Chinese practice of stimulating particular locations along the body's meridians to free the flow of energy (qi). Acupressure is another form of this treatment using hand pressure instead of needle punctures.

**analgesics.** Medications that relieve pain like nonsteroidals (aspirin), nonopioids (acetaminophen), or opioids (codeine).

**ankylosing spondylitis (AS).** An inflammatory arthritis of the spine associated with pain and stiffness that can result in the fusion (ankylosis) of the spinal joints and ligaments.

**annulus fibrosus.** The circular outer portion of the intervertebral disc.

**anti-inflammatory.** Reducing heat, swelling, pain, and loss of function.

**arachnoiditis.** Inflammation of the membrane surrounding the spinal cord. The most common cause is scarring from prior surgery. The scarring associated with this inflammation can cause chronic, persistent pain.

**arthritis.** Inflammation of a joint.

**biofeedback.** A method to use electronic instruments to generate data that is used to control bodily functions such as blood pressure, breathing, or heart rate.

**bisphosphonates.** A group of medicines utilized for treatment of osteoporosis that inhibit bone resorption by diminishing osteoclast function.

**bulging.** An outward swelling associated with mild flattening used to describe an intervertebral disc. Bulging does not have to cause nerve compression.

**bone mineral density (BMD).** The amount of calcium measured in a two dimensional space that helps determine risk for osteoporosis.

**C-reactive protein (CRP).** A protein produced by the liver that is increased in systemic inflammatory diseases.

**cauda equina.** The end of the spinal cord that starts at L1 and resembles the "tail of a horse."

**cervical.** Relating to the seven vertebrae in the neck between the skull and chest.

**claudication.** A cramping, burning, aching sensation in limbs brought on by activity that decreases blood flow to the nerves (neurogenic) or the muscles (vascular) supplying the extremity.

**coccydynia.** Pain in the coccyx usually related to a direct trauma falling on the buttock.

**coccyx.** The end of the spine, the tailbone. It is connected to the sacrum.

**computed axial tomography (CT).** A radiographic technique utilizing X rays and computer technology to visualize horizontal sections of the human body. Most useful for identifying bone abnormalities.

**conjunctivitis.** Inflammation of the superficial layer of the eye.

**conversion reaction.** Transformation of an emotion into a physical manifestation, hysteria.

**corticosteroids.** Hormones produced by the adrenal gland with properties to influence glucose metabolism and kidney function. A decrease in inflammation is a potential result of ingesting amounts greater than those produced by the adrenal gland on a daily basis.

**cryoablation.** The use of cold to freeze nerves to decrease pain particularly from facet joints.

**cyclooxygenase.** An enzyme that comes in two forms, I and II. Type I maintains body functions. Type II is associated with the development of inflammation. Aspirin inhibits I and II. COX-2 drugs inhibit type II only.

**degeneration.** A deterioration of tissues and cells that results in impairment or destruction of the structure.

**disc.** The cylinder-like structure composed of a gel center (nucleus pulposus) and a fibrous outer covering (annulus fibrosus) that acts as a shock absorber and a universal joint in the spine.

**discectomy.** Removal of all or part of an intervertebral disc.

**discitis.** Inflammation of the discs that may be an aseptic inflammation in children and an infection in adults.

**discography.** Radiographic visualization of the intervertebral disc space by injection of dye.

**dual energy X ray absorptiometry (DXA).** A method that uses two beams of X rays that measures the differences between soft tissues and bones to determine calcium content (see BMD).

**dura.** Membrane that surrounds the spinal cord and brain. Spinal fluid is contained within the dura.

**endorphins.** Naturally occurring pain-relieving chemicals produced during exercise and other physical activities.

**epidural.** A potential space between the dura and spinal column that is a frequent location for anti-inflammatory injections.

**erythrocyte sedimentation rate (ESR).** A test that measures the speed of the fall of clumped red blood cells in a tube. A fast fall rate corresponds to increased systemic inflammation.

**ergonomics.** The scientific study of the efficient use of the human body in work and recreation.

**extension.** In regard to the spine, bending backward.

**facet joints.** The paired joints located in the posterior portion of the vertebral bodies connecting the spine. These joints are part of the stabilizing mechanism for the spine.

**facet syndrome.** Irritation of a facet joint that may result in pain that radiates from the back down the leg.

**fascia.** A thin sheet of fibrous tissue enveloping muscles and structures below the skin.

**fibromyalgia.** A generalized musculoskeletal syndrome associated with tender points in specific locations on the body.

**flexion.** In regard to the spine, bending forward.

**fluoroscopy.** An X ray technique that allows for viewing of a moving body part.

**fusion.** In regard to the spine, a surgical procedure to unite two or more vertebrae with bone graft with or without metal supports resulting in immobilization of that portion. (Anterior interbody spinal fusion—procedure from the front of the spine with a disc space replaced with bone graft. Posterior interbody spinal fusion—procedure from the back of the spine with disc space replaced with bone graft. Posterior lateral spinal fusion—procedure from behind and from the side of the spinal column.)

**gadolinium.** The contrast material utilized with magnetic resonance imaging (MRI) to identify tissues with increased blood flow. Used to identify tumors, postsurgical scar tissue, and infections.

**gene.** The unit of a chromosome that transfers an inherited characteristic from parent to offspring.

**hamstring.** The muscles and tendons located in the back of the thigh.

**herniated disc.** Displacement of the central portion of an intervertebral disc (nucleus pulposus). The degrees of herniation include protrusion (gel contained within the annulus fibrosus), extrusion (gel displaced into the spinal canal beyond the annulus but remains connected to the central area), and sequestration (gel free and unattached to the original disc).

**inflammation.** A pathologic process associated with redness, heat, swelling, pain, and loss of function. This process destroys tissues but is also associated with the repair and healing of body structures.

**intervertebral.** Between two adjacent vertebrae.

**joint.** A specialized structure where two bones come in close proximity. The joint may facilitate movement (facet) or stability (sacroiliac) depending on the function of the joint.

**kyphosis.** A deformity of the spine associated with excessive forward bending, most commonly in the thoracic area.

**laminectomy.** A surgical procedure that removes a portion of the plate that serves as the back of the spinal canal. This decompression procedure is performed for treatment of herniated intervertebral discs and spinal stenosis.

**ligament.** A strong band of fibrous tissue connecting bones at a joint or holding organs in place.

**lordosis.** The forward curve located in the low back and neck.

**low back.** The area between the lower ribs and the lower crease of the buttocks.

**lumbar.** Relating to the five vertebrae between the chest and sacrum.

**magnetic resonance imaging (MRI).** A radiographic technique utilizing magnets and radio waves to visualize the internal structures of the human body. Overall, the most useful technique in the investigation of spinal abnormalities.

**manipulation.** Movement of the spine to restore normal function.

**muscle.** Specialized contractile tissue that generates force and facilitates movement.

**myelogram.** A radiographic technique where dye is injected into the spinal canal to better identify the spinal cord.

**narcotic.** A powerful pain-relieving drug associated with potential to cause significant alteration of mood and dependence following repeated administration. Opioids are narcotics.

**nerve.** Specialized cord-like tissue that transmits signals to and from the brain.

**neurotomy.** A procedure that destroys nerves supplying a structure. Heat or cold may be used to accomplish the goal of the procedure.

**nonsteroidal.** A medication that decreases inflammation that is not a corticosteroid.

**nucleus pulposus.** The gel center of the intervertebral disc. This is the portion of the disc that herniates.

**opioids.** Chemicals that bind to natural opioid receptors that promote analgesia. This group of chemicals include natural (derived from opium), semisynthetic (modified natural opioids), fully synthetic (manufactured), and endogenous (produced by our bodies).

**osteoarthritis.** The most common form of arthritis. The lumbar spine is a frequent location for this disorder. Osteophytes are bony projections that form on spinal joints in response to the changes of osteoarthritis.

**osteoporosis.** A disorder associated with decreased calcium in bone. This disorder is associated with increased risk of fracture in the spine (vertebrae), hip, and wrist.

**placebo.** An inert substance that is used in medical research to determine the degree of improvement that occurs by chance alone.

**qi.** The life energy that flows through body channels called meridians. A disease state is related to the imbalance of qi. Restoration of balanced flow to a healthy state can be achieved through acupuncture.

**rad.** A measure of radiation exposure. Normal background exposure to the sun during a year is about 0.6 rads.

**radiofrequency.** The generation of heat with the use of radio waves to damage nerves communicating pain signals particularly supplying facet joints (also called rhizotomy).

**radionuclide scan.** A radiographic test using a small amount of radioactive tracer that is injected intravenously. The tracer identifies tissues with abnormally increased activity. A bone scan is the test most frequently used to survey the entire spine for low back disorders.

**radiculopathy.** A disorder of the nerves after they exit the spine.

**reactive arthritis.** A disorder that causes conjunctivitis, urethritis, and arthritis. The lumbar spine and sacroiliac joints are injured in this disease.

**reflex.** An involuntary action that results from sensory input causing a muscular response.

**rheumatism.** Any ache or pain in the musculoskeletal system. Arthritis is a special form of rheumatism.

**sacrum.** Relating to the portion of the spine between the lumbar and coccyx. The sacroiliac joints connect the sacrum with the pelvis.

**sciatica.** A pain that follows the sciatic nerve down the leg to the calf or foot.

**scoliosis.** A lateral curvature of the spine.

**SERMs.** Selective estrogen receptor molecules work like estrogens to slow bone loss without hormone effects on the breast or uterus. They are used for treatment of osteoporosis.

**spinal cord.** The major nerve structure located within the spine that connects the brain with the rest of the human body.

**spinal stenosis.** A narrowing of the spinal canal resulting in compression of spinal nerves.

**spondyloarthropathy.** A group of disorders that causes inflammatory arthritis of the spine.

**spondylolisthesis.** An anterior displacement of a vertebra on the one below that can be the result of a spondylolysis that occurred during development as a teenager, or through degenerative changes in the facet joints.

**spondylolysis.** A defect in the growth plate between the joints in the back of a vertebra.

**spondylosis.** A degenerative disease of the discs and facet joints of the spine.

**strain.** An injury that occurs from overuse, frequently associated with muscles, fascia, and ligaments. The most common cause of mechanical low back pain in younger individuals.

**subluxation.** An abnormal movement or position of joint surfaces.

**syndrome.** A collection of complaints that together describe a disorder.

**tendon.** A tough, fibrous structure that attaches muscles to bones.

**thoracic.** Portion of the spine that contains the ribs between the cervical and lumbar regions of the spine.

**urethritis.** Inflammation of the lining of the urethra, the tube that connects the bladder with the surface of the body.

**vertebra.** One of the individual bones that form the spine. The shape and function of the vertebrae are specific to the different portions of the spine.

**X rays.** A form of electromagnetic energy that passes through an object, forming a charged particle that is imaged on a piece of film.

**yoga.** An Indian practice consisting of exercise, breathing, and meditation that improves balance and posture.

# Appendix A

# Dr. B's Back School FAQ

IN THE LATE 1960S, a Swedish physical therapist, Marianne Zachrisson-Forssell, developed a sound-slide program that included basic information about low back pain. The four one-hour sessions included information on anatomy and function of the spine, body mechanics, and exercise programs. The classes also included question-and-answer sessions to address any issues that were not addressed during the slide lectures.

The enthusiasm for back schools in the United States slowly increased over time. Physicians, physical therapists, and nurse specialists teach the courses. Back schools exist in medical schools, community hospitals, YMCAs, and industrial settings.

The methods of teaching vary at back schools depending on the philosophy of the organizers. "Students" may be given classroom instruction, or demonstrations of exercises and work habits, or motivation. Teaching methods vary around the world. The Swedish Back School is designed as a general information program with an exercise program to improve physical conditioning. The Canadian Back School uses psychological approaches to increase self-awareness about pain and function. The role of anxiety and stress is emphasized. The California Back School teaches how to control acute low back pain. Individuals go through an obstacle course to measure physical function. Instruction over a three-week period improves physical function.

Do back schools help people prevent recurrences of back pain? A study was conducted in a Volvo car plant where back school instruction was matched against back exercises or heat therapy. Employees who attended back school had fewer days off work than the other two groups.

When I was the director of the Spine Center at the local medical center, I helped organize their back school. A number of back pain sufferers became students at the school. The instructors of the classes had an opportunity to compile a number of questions that were repeatedly asked at the back school sessions. Here are some of the most frequently asked questions and my most current answers.

**Is any particular chair helpful for low back pain?**
It depends on the location of the chair: at work, at home, or in the car. Is the chair to prevent pain or to treat pain? There's no one chair for all locations and situations.

In the acute low back pain situation, the very stable, firm chair is best. The chair should have a small amount of cushioning for comfort. The area on the surface of the seat should allow some movement of the legs. The chair seat should not be too low, causing your legs to be close to your chest. Legs should be at ninety degrees or slightly higher than your hips if you prefer a flat back. The back of the chair should have a slight angle. Armrests decrease pressure on your low back.

A variety of lumbar lordosis seat supports are available. Some pillows are made of foam, while some are inflatable. See if you would benefit from a seat support by rolling up a towel and putting it around your waist. If the addition of the towel decreases your pain, you should consider a seat support. The support can be used on the chair at work and in the car.

Designers of new car models realize the importance of seat supports and have built adjustments into the seat in the car that can be altered for comfort. Do not be afraid to try different positions of the seat to try to maximize comfort. Other car seats are too soft for comfort when you have back pain. The lack of support makes the muscles of the back work constantly, causing increased spasm and pain. A support for the back of the car seat may be adequate if the seat bottom offers adequate stability. If the seat is too soft, a single support that includes a seat bottom and back is useful.

Some of my patients have had so much concern about buying a car because of the issue of the seats that I have suggested that they rent a car. Not just any car, but the model they plan to buy. They can determine if the adjustments of the seat make their commutes tolerable. Hopefully you will not need to rent too many to get the car and the seat you like.

A number of recliners are available with a variety of adjustments for comfort. I believe these chairs to be more comfortable when you are rehabilitating from your back attack as opposed to being in the middle of one. The amount of cushioning, the degree of reclining, and massage and heat attachments are matters of personal preference. None of these factors are particularly helpful in preventing back pain. If they make you feel better and the price is in your budget, you should pamper yourself.

When talking about the office, not all your work has to be done while you are seated. In fact, for some people with leg pain, a standing work desk can offer comfort at work. A forty-eight-year-old attorney came to my office because of increasing pain while at work. He'd had a cervical and lumbar spine operation within the last four years, and he had a recurrence of leg pain that was responding to conservative management. His greatest problem was long hours at work and during conferences. He had tried a number of chairs, but none would allow him to work for any length of time. I suggested that he obtain a standing work desk and use that whenever his leg became painful. I also suggested that he stand more at conferences. The combination helped calm his leg pain over the next six months. He became so fond of his standing desk that he kept on using it even after his leg pain resolved.

The bottom line is try out any seat, recliner, cushion, massager, corset, or support before you make a purchase, do not go by reputation alone.

### Does inversion boot therapy help back pain?

Regular traction has not been shown to be helpful for low back or leg pain on a consistent basis. Traction used to be a way to get patients to stay in bed in the hospital. But we know now that bed rest for longer than two days is not helpful for low back pain. Traction of the lumbar spine is not a recommended therapy.

But what about inversion boots? You know, hanging upside down like a bat with your feet attached to boots with clips that hang from a bar, or a table that rotates your entire body. The thought behind these techniques is that the weight of your body will spread out the disc space allowing for displaced disc material to return to its normal position. Unfortunately, no studies are available that show that these techniques work to reverse herniated discs. In addition, there are real life-threatening events associated with inversion therapy.

First, I never understood how people with back pain were going to be able to attach their boots to the bar. And more importantly, how were they going to get themselves down. Second, being inverted causes increased pressure in the eyes. Detached retinas are associated with inversion therapy. Third, you should know if aneurysms (weakening of blood vessels) are a family trait. Individuals with berry aneurysms have had bleeding into the brain with inverted positions since this increases blood pressure to the head. Finally, the bar holding the boots must be attached appropriately. Individuals have become quadriplegic when they have fractured their necks when falling to the ground. For all these reasons, inversion therapy is not recommended for back pain.

### Do my high heel shoes cause back pain?

Sometimes. High heel shoes raise you off the ground, tending to shift your center of gravity. In response to this new position, you may bend backward to stay in balance. The higher the heel, the greater is the apparent sway in the back. If bending backward on dry land makes your back feel worse, so will high heels. A compromise may be shoes that are between flats and full high heels. They do not cause as much of a change in the shape of the spine and may be acceptable from a fashion point of view. The other possibility when wearing a higher heel is limiting the time you stand in them and doing pelvic tilt exercises to flatten your spine when the opportunity allows.

### Does prolotherapy help low back pain?

Prolotherapy is an injection therapy. An irritation solution of glucose, glycerine, or phenol is injected into tissue of the back. The fluids start a healing response to reverse the instability of the spine or surrounding joints, including the sacroiliac.

Studies have suggested that injections into spinal tissues with or without irritating fluids result in improvement. It may be the injection and the interaction with the physician as opposed to what is injected that really counts.

Some individuals have a reaction to the injected fluids with persistent pain. Prolotherapy is not always benign. I have had some individuals who are hypermobile try prolotherapy with the hope that scarring will result in decreased motion. They heal with scar tissues that includes as much elastic fibers as their normal tissues. In general, I have not found this therapy to be better than a simple injection with anesthetic.

**What does the circular that comes with my prescription drug package mean? It scares me half to death.**

The package circular is the information supplied by the drug manufacturer that is required by the FDA. It contains basic information about the drug, including all the possible side effects and drug interactions.

The information regarding the potential side effects of a drug is generated during the clinical trials studying the efficacy of the agent. As a clinical investigator, I have had personal experience with the information gathered during these trials. If any change occurs during the study, that information is considered an adverse event. This information is counted during the study and the final number is listed in the package circular.

Anything is possible, but the side effects that occur frequently are really the only ones to be concerned about. For example, in one package circular that I reviewed, food poisoning was listed as a possible side effect. Obviously, someone taking part in the study went to a restaurant and had a bad meal. Even though that had nothing to do with the study drug, that happening was considered an adverse event. This kind of information dilutes the value of this important source of information for patients and doctors.

Remember the package circular lists problems that may happen. You may experience none of them. However, if you become aware of some interaction, tell your doctor immediately, so he or she can decide if the medicine is the best one to improve your condition.

**How about Botox injections for my back spasm?**

Clostridium botulinum bacteria produce a toxin that is a powerful paralyzing agent. Botulism is the life-threatening illness associated with ingestion of contaminated food. When injected in small amounts, the toxin reverses muscle spasms. The muscles are not able to contract for as long as four months after an injection. Botox is the brand name of the purified form of botulinum toxin.

The injections have benefits and risks. The injection will relieve muscle contractions and will resolve associated myalgias. The risks are associated with rare, but serious reactions including difficulty breathing and swallowing. Also the paralysis of a muscle for an extended period of time does not improve its function. The injections are expensive.

I have not recommended these injections for my patients.

**Which is the best aerobic exercise machine for a person with back pain?**

A gym will offer a choice of cardiovascular exercise machines from rowing machines to elliptical trainers. Many of my patients ask which one to try. The choices include a treadmill, elliptical trainer, stationary bicycle, stair climber, and rowing machine. The assumption is that you will use the equipment appropriately. Any machine can cause a problem if you use it incorrectly.

I believe that the stationary bicycle is my first choice. The bicycle can be upright or recumbent. There is low impact. The elevation of the seat can be altered as necessary for comfort.

Rowing machines can be a real problem if you bend too far forward or backward. Keeping a straight back can help prevent potential for injury.

I usually recommend upright machines (treadmill, bicycle) as you have almost resolved your episode of back pain. Remember the Comfort Zone. Start slow and build up your time and distance.

**Can I go horseback riding?**

Many of my patients love to ride their horses as much as possible. Being my patients, they have visited me for evaluation and treatment of their pain. Their goal was always to get back to riding. The variety of complaints have spanned from simple muscles aches, disc herniations, and sciatica, to persistent back pain after two back surgeries.

Studies have attempted to answer the question "Does horseback riding cause degeneration of the spine?" Reassuring to horseback riders is the answer *no*! Studies have shown that equestrians, independent of riding discipline (jumping, dressage), have no greater changes in spinal parts than those nonriding individuals. In general, however, horseback riders do have more back pain than the average population.

My recommendations include a period of time without riding to determine if riding is playing a major role in causing persistence of the pain. Appropriate components of the basic back pain relief program are instituted. The program includes exercises to strengthen the core muscles surrounding the spine. Riding is resumed as pain is reduced. The duration of riding is gradually increased so that the rides do not become excessively fatiguing.

I have to say that these patients are my most dedicated to getting better. They follow instructions and try to improve as rapidly as possible. I try to remind them that using excellent riding technique and not falling from their horses is a great way of staying in the saddle. The double meaning of this statement is something that they readily agree with.

**What sports can I safely play if I have back pain?**
In the acute stage of back pain, limiting sports activities is appropriate. Movement is important, but shooting eighteen holes is not going to be helpful. Allowing your back to heal will actually allow you to return and stay functional as opposed to going back too soon and having recurrent attacks stretching out your recovery.

Sport activities can be divided into low, moderate, and high risk for developing low back pain. If you have back pain and are trying to start a new sport, you should speak with your physician before starting a new activity. In general, some of the low-risk sports are compatible with low back pain. These sports are bicycling and swimming. Racquet sports are difficult to start if you are having acute back pain. Also, I have assumed that amateur sports persons are involved with these activities. Professional athletes have greater risks.

- Low-risk sports: bicycling, hockey, skiing, soccer, squash, swimming, tennis
- Moderate-risk sports: baseball, basketball, bowling, some types of dancing, golf, horseback riding, jogging, rowing
- High-risk sports: diving, football, gymnastics, weight lifting

The low-risk sports in general put little pressure on the spine. In addition, the risk of continuous twisting is small. The moderate-risk sports are associated with jumping (basketball, dancing, horseback riding, jogging) or twisting (baseball, bowling, golf, rowing). Jumping places increased pressures on discs. Discs are at risk of herniation or more rapid degeneration. Twisting places pressure on the facet joints. Continuous twisting causes increased joint pain that continues after the sports activity is completed. High-risk sports are associated with high velocity impact (diving, football) or hyperextension (gymnastics) or excessive weight (lifting).

General recommendations for all sports are to use good technique from the outset. You should learn from a good teacher if you have not had experience with the sport. You should ask a ski instructor about appropriate technique to protect your back. You should use appropriate equipment to decrease your exposure to risk. For example, good running shoes with appropriate cushioning are important. Running on soft surfaces like grass or asphalt is better than running on concrete.

**Can I play golf without increasing my back pain?**
Low back pain problems are the most frequent injury in amateur golfers. This problem also occurs frequently in professional golfers. Golf injuries occur from overuse and develop over time. Amateur golfers are at risk because they play sporadically, without proper warm-up, and have less-than-ideal swing mechanics. Overpracticing poor mechanics increases the risk of injury.

The golf swing results in the riskiest motions for your spine—a hyperextension and rotation. Back pain results from the rotation of the spine in the back swing, and hyperextension in the follow-through. These motions place many times the golfer's body weight across the lower discs of the lumbar spine.

Back problems can be prevented if appropriate care is given to preparation and appropriate technique. It is imperative that golfers warm up for at least ten minutes and include the following:

*Stretching (two minutes)*
- Neck rotations
- Shoulder stretch
- Trunk side bends
- Trunk rotation
- Toe touches (sitting on bench)

*Driving range (three minutes)*
- Half swing—sand wedge
- Three-quarter swing—5 iron
- Full swing—driver

*Putting (four minutes)*
- Back-and-forth putting green
- Waiting to tee off (one minute)
- Practice swings
- Visualize good form

When in doubt, consider lessons from the golf professional to perfect your swing. Appropriate warm-up and good technique are the best ways to decrease overrotation and hyperextension that increase the risk for low back injuries.

# Appendix B

## *Medications for Low Back Pain*

| Trade Name (Chemical Class) | Dosage (mg) | Frequency (times/day) | Half-life (hours) | Comment |
|---|---|---|---|---|
| **NSAIDs** | | | | |
| Anaprox (naproxen sodium) | 275/550 | 3–4 | 13 | OTC brand is Aleve |
| Ansaid (flurbiprofen) | 50/100 | 2–3 | 6 | long-acting ibuprofen |
| Arthrotec (diclofenac/misoprostol) | 50/75 | 2–3 | 2 | prevents stomach ulcers |
| Ascriptin (aspirin + antacid) | 325 | 4–6 | 4 | inexpensive |
| Bayer (aspirin) | 325 | 4–6 | 4 | rapid onset of action |
| Cataflam (diclofenac potassium) | 25/50 | 2–3 | 2 | less risk of ulcers (COX-2) |
| Celebrex (celecoxib) | 50/100/200/400 | 2 | 11 | |
| Clinoril (sulindac) | 150/200 | 2 | 18 | |
| Daypro (oxaprozin) | 600 | 1–2 | 25 | once-a-day convenience |
| Disalcid (salsalate) | 500/750 | 2 | 4 | |
| Dolobid (diflunisal) | 250/500 | 2–3 | 11 | |
| Easprin (enteric-coated aspirin) | 975 | 4 | 4 | less GI upset |
| Ecotrin (enteric-coated aspirin) | 325 | 4–6 | 4 | less GI upset |
| Feldene (piroxicam) | 10/20 | 1 | 38–45 | long-acting |
| Flector (diclofenac patch) | 2 | 2 | | patch over painful area |
| Indocin (indomethacin) | 50–100 | 1–3 | 4 | for spondyloarthropathy |
| Lodine (etodolac) | 200–500 | 2–4 | 6 | |
| Meclomen (meclofenamate) | 50/100 | 4 | 4 | |
| Mobic (meloxicam) | 7.5/15 | 1 | 15 | like COX-2 drug |
| Motrin (ibuprofen) | 200/400/800 | 4–6 | 1–3 | requires large doses |
| Nalfon (fenoprofen) | 200/300 | 3–4 | 2–3 | more kidney irritation |
| Naprelan (naproxen) | 375/500/750 | 1 | 13 | OTC brand is Aleve |
| Naprosyn (naproxen) | 250/375/500 | 3 | 13 | |

| Drug | Dose | | | Comments |
|---|---|---|---|---|
| Orudis (ketoprofen) | 25–75 | 3–4 | 3–4 | |
| Oruvail (ketoprofen) | 200 | 1 | 3–4 | extended release form |
| Pennsaid (diclofenac solution) | 4 | 2 | | contains DMSO |
| Ponstel (mefenamic acid) | 250 | 4 | 4 | |
| Relafen (nabumetone) | 500/750 | 2 | 2–6 | less GI distress |
| Tolectin (tolmetin) | 200/400 | 4 | 4 | |
| Toradol (ketorolac) | 10 | 4 | 4–6 | analgesic, but ulcer risk |
| Trilisate (choline magnesium trisalicylate) | 500/750 | 2 | 4 | |
| Voltaren (diclofenac sodium) | 25–100 | 2–3 | 2 | |
| Voltaren (diclofenac gel) | 4 | 2 | | up to 32 gm per day |
| Zorprin (time–release aspirin) | 800 | 2 | 4 | less GI upset |
| **NONOPIOID ANALGESICS** | | | | |
| Lidoderm (lidocaine) | 5% | 1 | 2 | 3 patches maximum |
| Ryzolt (tramadol) | 100/200/300 | 1 | 4 | slow release |
| Tylenol (acetaminophen) | 325/500/650 | 3 | 4 | |
| Ultracet (tramadol/acetaminophen) | 37.5/325 | 4 | 4 | requires frequent doses |
| Ultram (tramadol) | 50 | 4 | 4 | requires frequent doses |
| Ultram ER (tramadol) | 100/200/300 | 1 | 4 | slow release |
| **OPIOID ANALGESICS** | | | | |
| Avinza (morphine) | 30/45/60/75/90/120 | 1 | 4 | slow release |
| Codeine (codeine) | 15–60 | 4–6 | 4 | frequent GI distress |
| Darvocet (propoxyphene/acetaminophen) | 50/65/100 | 4 | 12/35 | acetaminophen 325 mg/650 mg |
| Darvon (propoxyphene) | 65 | 4 | 12/35 | prolonged half–life in elderly |

(continued)

| Trade Name (Chemical Class) | Dosage (mg) | Frequency (times/day) | Half-life (hours) | Comment |
|---|---|---|---|---|
| Darvon Compound (propoxyphene/aspirin) | 32/65 | 4 | 12/35 | aspirin 389 mg |
| Darvon-N (propoxyphene) | 100 | 4 | 12/35 | frequent interactions |
| Demerol (meperidine) | 50/100 | 6 | 3 | |
| Dilaudid (hydromorphone) | 2/3/8 | 4 | 3 | |
| Duragesic (fentanyl) | 25–100 (mcg) | 1 | 17 | topical every 3 days |
| Embeda (morphine/naltrexone) | 20–100/0.8–4 | 3 | 79 | withdrawal if chewed |
| Fentora (fentanyl) | 100/200/400/600/800 (mcg) | 4 | 4 | quick-acting |
| Kadian (morphine) | 20–100 | 1 | 4 | slow release |
| Lortab (hydrocodone/acetaminophen) | 2.5/7.5/10 | 4 | 4 | acetaminophen 500 mg |
| Methadone | 5/10/40 | 3 | 60 | chronic pain |
| MS Contin (morphine) | 15–200 | 2 | 4 | slow release |
| Nucynta (tapentadol) | 50/75/100 | 4 | 4 | less constipation |
| Opana/ER (oxymorphone) | 5/7.5/10/15/20/30/40 | 2 | 11 | immediate/slow release |
| Oxycodone | 5 | 4 | 3 | immediate form |
| OxyContin (oxycodone) | 10–80 | 2 | 5 | slow release |
| Percocet (oxycodone/acetaminophen) | 2.5–10 | 4 | 4 | acetaminophen 325 mg/650 mg |
| Percodan (oxycodone/aspirin) | 4.5 | 4 | 4 | aspirin 325 mg |
| Tylenol #2/3/4 (codeine/acetaminophen) | 15–60 | 4 | 4 | acetaminophen 325 mg |
| Vicodin (hydrocodone/acetaminophen) | 5–10 | 4 | 4 | acetaminophen 325 mg/750 mg |
| Vicoprofen (hydrocodone/ibuprofen) | 7.5 | 4 | 4 | ibuprofen 200 mg |
| Xodol (hydrocodone/acetaminophen) | 5/7.5/10 | 4 | 4 | acetaminophen 300 mg |

**MUSCLE RELAXANTS**

| | | | | |
|---|---|---|---|---|
| Amrix (cyclobenzaprine) | 15/30 | 1 | 8–37 | less sleepiness |
| Dantrium (dantrolene) | 25/50/100 | 4 | 9 | spasticity |
| Fexmid (cyclobenzaprine) | 7.5 | 1–3 | 8 | |
| Flexeril (cyclobenzaprine) | 5/10 | 1–3 | 8–37 | sleepiness, a toxicity |
| Lioresal (baclofen) | 10/20 | 3 | 4 | spasticity |
| Norflex (ophenadrine) | 100 | 2 | 8 | |
| Parafon (chlorzoxazone) | 250/500 | 4 | 4 | |
| Robaxin (methocarbamol) | 500/750 | 4 | 2 | |
| Skelaxin (metaxalone) | 800 | 4 | 3 | |
| Soma (carisoprodol) | 250/350 | 4 | 4–6 | addictive properties |
| Valium (diazepam) | 2/5/10 | 4 | 24 | withdrawal problems |
| Zanaflex (tizanidine) | 2/4/6 | 3 | 8 | spasticity |

# Appendix C

# *Best Back Resources*

## ORGANIZATIONS AND WEBSITES

Heal Your Back/Back in Control Website: www.drborenstein.com
This website contains references for this book. Updated information
on FAQ and patient profiles added on a regular basis.

American College of Rheumatology (ACR)
2200 Lake Boulevard NE
Atlanta, GA 30319
Phone: (404) 633-3777
Website: www.rheumatology.org
The national professional organization of rheumatologists

Arthritis Foundation (AF)
1330 West Peachtree Street
Atlanta, GA 30309
Website: www.arthritis.org
The national organization for the support of individuals with all forms
of arthritis

American Academy of Orthopaedic Surgeons (AAOS)
6300 N. River Road
Rosemont, IL 60018-4262
Phone: (800) 346-2267
Website: www.aaos.org
The national professional organization of orthopedic surgeons

American Osteopathic Association (AOA)
142 East Ontario Street
Chicago, IL 60611
Phone: (800) 621-1773
Website: www.osteopathic.org
The national professional organization of osteopathic physicians


American Physical Therapy Association (APTA)
1111 North Fairfax Street
Alexandria, VA 22314
Phone: (800) 999-2782
Website: www.apta.org
The national professional organization for physical therapists


American Chiropractic Association (ACA)
1701 Clarendon Boulevard
Arlington, VA 22209
Phone: (800) 986-4636
Website: www.acatoday.org
The national professional organization of chiropractors


American Massage Therapy Association (AMTA)
500 Davis Street, Suite 900
Evanston, IL 60201
Phone: (847) 864-0123
Website: www.amtamassage.org
The national professional organization for massage therapists


National Library of Medicine
Website: www.nlm.nih.gov


American Yoga Association
P.O. Box 19986
Sarasota, FL 34276
Phone (941) 927-4977
Website: www.americanyoga association.org

National Institutes of Health
Bethesda, MD 20892
Phone: (301) 496-4000
Website: www.nih.gov

National Center for Complementary and Alternative Medicine
Website: www.nccam.nih.gov

Agency for Healthcare Research and Quality (AHRQ)
Website: www.ahrq.gov

Food and Drug Administration
Website: www.fda.gov

Spondylitis Association of America
P.O. Box 5872
Sherman Oaks, CA 91413
Phone: (800) 777-8189
Website: www.spondylitis.org

National Center for Homeopathy (NCH)
801 North Fairfax Street, Suite 306
Alexandria, VA 22314
Phone: (703) 548-7790
Website: www.nationalcenterforhomeopathy.org

U.S. Pilates Association (USPA)
Website: www.pilates-studio.com

## PUBLICATIONS

Bigos SJ, Bowyer O, Braen G, et al. *Acute Low Back Problems in Adults.*
Clinical Practice Guideline No. 14. AHCPR Publication No. 95-0642.
Rockville, MD: Agency for Health Care Policy and Research, Pub-
lic Health Service, U.S. Department of Health and Human Services,
December 1994.
Borenstein DG, Wiesel SW, Boden SD. *Low Back and Neck Pain: Com-
prehensive Diagnosis and Management.* Philadelphia: W. B. Saunders,
2004.

Horstman J. *The Arthritis Foundation's Guide to Alternative Therapies.* Atlanta: Arthritis Foundation, 1999.

Jellin JM (ed). *Natural Medicine: Comprehensive Database.* Stockton: Therapeutic Research Faculty, 2010. (Available in book, PDA, or web versions.)

Inclusion of websites and publications in this appendix does not imply approval of their content.

# References

## CHAPTER 1: UNDERSTANDING WHY YOUR BACK HURTS

Andersson GBJ. The epidemiology of spinal disorders. In: Frymoyer JW, ed. *The Adult Spine: Principles and Practice*, 2nd ed. New York: Raven Press; 1997:93–133.

Borenstein DG, Wiesel SW, Boden SD. *Low Back and Neck Pain: Comprehensive Diagnosis and Management*, 3rd ed. Philadelphia: Saunders; 2004:921.

Harrison PJ, Tunbridge EM. Catechol-O-methyltransferase (COMT): a gene contributing to sex differences in brain function, and to sexual dimorphism in the predisposition to psychiatric disorders. *Neuropsychopharmacology*. 2008;33:3037–3045.

Lawrence RC, Felson DT, Helmick CG, et al. Estimates of the prevalence of arthritis and other rheumatic conditions in the United States. Part II. *Arthritis Rheum*. 2008;58:26–35.

Siddall PJ, Cousins MJ. Spine Update: Spinal pain mechanisms. *Spine*. 1997;22:98–104.

## CHAPTER 2: WORKING WITH YOUR DOCTOR

Chou R, Qaseem A, Snow V, et al. Diagnosis and treatment of low back pain: A joint clinical practice guideline from the American College of Physicians and the American Pain Society. *Ann Intern Med*. 2007;147:478–491.

Deyo RA, Rainville J, Kent DL. What can the history and physical examination tell us about low back pain? *JAMA*. 1992;268:760–765.

## CHAPTER 3: WHAT DIAGNOSTIC TESTS CAN— AND CANNOT—TELL YOU

Boden SD, David DO, Dina TS, et al. Abnormal magnetic resonance scans of the lumbar spine in asymptomatic subjects: A prospective investigation. *J Bone Joint Surg Am*. 1990;72:403–408.

Borenstein DG, O'Mara JW Jr, Boden SD, et al. The value of magnetic resonance imaging of the lumbar spine to predict low back pain in asymptomatic subjects. A seven-year follow-up study. *J Bone Joint Surg Am.*
2001;83:1306–1311.

Carragee EJ, Don AS, Hurwitz EL, et al. 2009 ISSLS Prize Winner: Does discography cause accelerated progression of degeneration changes in the
lumbar disc: A ten-year matched cohort study. *Spine.* 2009;34:2338–2345.

Carragee EJ, Lincoln T, Parmar VS, et al. A gold standard evaluation of the
"discogenic pain" diagnosis as determined by provocative discography.
*Spine.* 2006;31:2115–2123.

Gilbert JW, Wheeler GR, Lingreen RA, et al. Imaging in the position that
causes pain. *Surg Neurol.* 2008;69:463–465.

Leslie WD, Lix LM, Tsang JF, et al. Single-site vs. multisite bone density measurement for fracture prediction. *Arch Intern Med.* 2007;167:1641–1647.

Madsen R, Jensen TS, Pope M, et al. The effect of body position and axial
load on spinal canal morphology: An MRI study of central spinal stenosis.
*Spine.* 2008;33:61–67.

Smith-Bindman R, Lipson J, Marcus R, et al. Radiation dose associated with
common computed tomography examinations and the associated lifetime
attributable risk of cancer. *Arch Intern Med.* 2009;169:2078–2086.

## CHAPTER 4: THE BASIC BACK PAIN RELIEF PROGRAM

Bergholdt K, Fabricius RN, Bendix T. Better backs by better beds? *Spine.*
2008;33:703–708.

Cherkin DC, Deyo RA, Battie M, et al. A comparison of physical therapy, chiropractic manipulation, and provision of an educational booklet for the
treatment of patients with low back pain. *N Engl J Med..* 1998;339:1021–
1029.

Chou R, Atlas SJ, Stanos SP, et al. Nonsurgical interventional therapies for low
back pain: A review of the evidence for an American Pain Society Clinical
Practice Guideline. *Spine.* 2009;34:1078–1093.

Deyo RA, Diehl AK, Rosenthal M. How many days of bed rest for acute low
back pain? A randomized clinical trial. *N Engl J Med..* 1986;315:1064–1070.

Harper CM, Lyles YM. Physiology and complications of bed rest. *J Am Geriatr
Soc.* 1988;36:1047–1054.

Kovacs FM, Abraira V, Pena A, et al. Effect of firmness of mattress on chronic
non-specific low-back pain: Randomised, double-blind, controlled, mul-
ticentre trial. *Lancet.* 2003;362:1599–1604.

Landen BR. Heat or cold for the relief of low back pain? *Phys Ther.*
1967;47:1126–1128.

Malmivarra A, Hakkinen U, Aro T, et al. The treatment of acute low back pain:
Bed rest, exercises, or ordinary activity? *N Engl J Med..* 1995;351–355.

Million R, Nilsen KH, Jayson MIV, et al. Evaluation of low back pain and assessment of lumbar corsets with and without back supports. *Ann Rheum Dis.* 1981;40:449–454.

Roelofs P, Bierma-Zeinstra SMA, van Poppel MNM, et al. Lumbar supports to prevent recurrent low back pain among home care workers: A randomized trial. *Ann Intern Med.* 2007;147:685–692.

## CHAPTER 5: RECOGNIZING AND TREATING MECHANICAL LOW BACK PAIN

Atlas SJ, Delitto A. Spinal stenosis: Surgical versus nonsurgical treatment. *Clin Orthop Rel Res.* 2006;31:254–259.

Beurkens AJ, de Vet HC, Koke AJ, et al. Efficacy of traction for nonspecific low back pain: 12-week and 6-month results of a randomized clinical trial. *Spine.* 1997;22:2756–2762.

Beutler WJ, Frederickson BE, Murtland A, et al. The natural history of spondylolysis and spondylolisthesis: 45-year follow-up evaluation. *Spine.* 2003;28:1027–1035.

Borenstein DG, Korn S. Efficacy of a low-dose regimen of cyclobenzaprine hydrochloride in acute skeletal muscle spasm: Results of two placebo-controlled trials. *Clin Ther.* 2003;25:1056–1073.

Botwin KP, Gruber RD. Lumbar epidural steroid injections in the patient with lumbar spinal stenosis. *Phys Med Rehabil Clin N Am.* 2003;14:121–141.

Bradford DS, Tay B, Hu S. Adult scoliosis: Surgical indications, operative management, complications, and outcomes. *Spine.* 1999;24:2617–2629.

Chou R, Loeser JD, Owens DK, et al. Interventional therapies, surgery, and interdisciplinary rehabilitation for low back pain: An evidence-based clinical practice guideline from the American Pain Society. *Spine.* 2009;34:1066–1077.

Kelly J. Save yourself and back of the snow-clearing heroics. *Washington Post,* December 22, 2009.

Kirschner JS, Foye PM, Cole JL. Piriformis syndrome, diagnosis and treatment. *Muscle Nerve.* 2009;40:10–18.

Malanga GA, Ruoff GE, Weil AJ, et al. Cyclobenzaprine ER for muscle spasm associated with low back and neck pain: Two randomized, double-blind, placebo-controlled studies of identical design. *Curr Med Res Opin.* 2009;25:1179–1196.

Mariconda M, Galasso O, Secondulfo V, et al. Minimum 25-year outcome and functional assessment of lumbar discectomy. *Spine.* 2006;31:2593–2599.

Moller H, Hedlund R. Surgery versus conservative management in adult isthmic spondylolisthesis: A prospective randomized study. *Spine.* 2000;25:1711–1715.

North RB, Han M, Zahurak M, et al. Radiofrequency lumbar facet denervation: Analysis of prognostic factors. *Pain.* 1994;57:77–83.

Porter RW. Spinal stenosis and neurogenic claudication. *Spine.* 1996;21:2046–2052.

Weinstein JN, Lurie JD, Tosteson TD, et al. Surgical versus nonoperative treatment for lumbar disc herniation: Four-year results for the Spine Patient Outcomes Research Trial (SPORT). *Spine.* 2008;33:2789–2800.

## CHAPTER 6: RECOGNIZING AND TREATING
## MEDICAL CAUSES OF LOW BACK PAIN

Abrahm JL, Banffy MB, Harris MB. Spinal cord compression in patients with advanced metastatic cancer. *JAMA.* 2008;299:937–946.

Borenstein D. Prevalence and treatment outcome of primary and secondary fibromyalgia in patients with spinal pain. *Spine.* 1995;20:796–800.

Carragee EJ. Pyogenic vertebral osteomyelitis. *J Bone Joint Surg Am.* 1997;79:874–880.

Darouiche RO. Spinal epidural abscess. *N Engl J Med.* 2006;355:2012–2020.

David JC, van der Heijde DM, Braun J, et al. Sustained durability and tolerability of Etanercept in ankylosing spondylitis for 96 weeks. *Ann Rheum Dis.* 2005;64:1557–1562.

Hauser W, Petzke F, Sommer C. Comparative efficacy and harms of duloxetine, milnacipran, and pregabalin in fibromyalgia syndrome. *J Pain.* 2010;11:505–521.

Inman RD, David JC Jr, Heijde D, et al. Efficacy and safety of golimumab in patients with ankylosing spondylitis: Results of a randomized, double-blind, placebo-controlled, phase III trial. *Arthritis Rheum.* 2008;58:3402–3412.

Khan MA. An overview of clinical spectrum and heterogeneity of spondyloarthropathies. *Rheum Dis Clin N Am.* 1992;18:1–10.

Ostgaard HC, Zetherstrom G, Roos-Hansson E, et al. Reduction of back and posterior pelvic pain in pregnancy. *Spine.* 1994;19:894–900.

Van der Heijde D, Dijkmans B, Geusens P, et al. Efficacy and safety of Infliximab in patients with ankylosing spondylitis: Results of a randomized, placebo-controlled trial (ASSERT). *Arthritis Rheum.* 2005;52:582–591.

Van der Heijde D, Kivitz A, Schiff MH, et al. Efficacy and safety of adalimumab in patients with ankylosing spondylitis: Results of a multicenter, randomized, double-blind, placebo-controlled trial. *Arthritis Rheum.* 2006;54:2136–2146.

Weyand CM, Fulbright JW, Evans JM, et al. Corticosteroid requirements in polymyalgia rheumatica. *Arch Intern Med.* 1999;159:577–584.

Wolfe F, Clauw DJ, Fitzcharles M, et al. The American College of Rheumatology preliminary diagnostic criteria for fibromyalgia and measurement of symptom severity. *Arthritis Care Res.* 2010;62:600–610.

Bischoff-Ferrari HA, Willett WC, Wong JB. Fracture prevention with vitamin D supplementation: A meta-analysis of randomized controlled trials. *JAMA.* 2005;293: 2257–2264.

Black DM, Delmas PD, Eastell R, et al. Once-yearly zolendronic acid for treatment of postmenopausal osteoporosis. *N Engl J Med.* 2007;356:1809–1822.

Black DM, Schwartz AV, Ensrud KE, et al. Effects of continuing or stopping alendronate after years of treatment: The Fracture Intervention Trial Long-term Extension (FLEX): a randomized trial. *JAMA.* 2006;296:2927–2938.

Bone HG, Hosking D, Devogelaer J, et al. Ten years' experience with alendronate for osteoporosis in postmenopausal women. *N Engl J Med.* 2004;350:1189–1199.

Cauley JA, Hochberg MC, Lui L, et al. Long-term risk of incident vertebral fractures. *JAMA.* 2007;298:2761–2767.

Cauley JA, Robbins J, Chen Z, et al. Effects of estrogen plus progestin on risk of fracture and bone mineral density. The women's health initiative randomized trial. *JAMA.* 2003;290:1729–1738.

Chestnut CH III, Silverman S, Andriano K, et al. A randomized trial of nasal spray salmon Calcitonin in postmenopausal women with established osteoporosis: The Prevent Recurrence of Osteoporotic Fracture study. *Am J Med.* 2000;102:267–276.

Delmas PD, Ensrud KE, Adachi JD, et al. Efficacy of raloxifene on vertebral fracture risk reduction in postmenopausal women with osteoporosis: Four-year results from a randomized clinical trial. *J Clin Endocrinol Metab.* 2002;87:3609–3617.

Ebeling PR. Osteoporosis in men. *N Engl J Med.* 2008;358:1474–1482.

Greenspan SL, Bone HG, Ettinger MP, et al. Effect of recombinant human parathyroid hormone (1–84) on vertebral fracture and bone mineral density in postmenopausal women with osteoporosis: A randomized trial. *Ann Inter Med.* 2007;146:326–339.

Holick MF. Vitamin D deficiency. *N Engl J Med.* 2007;357:266–281.

Kanis JA, Johnell O, Oden A, et al. FRAX and the assessment of fracture probability in men and women from the UK. *Osteoporo Int.* 2008;19:385–397.

McClung MR, Lewiecki EM, Cohen SB, et al. Denosumab in postmenopausal women with low bone mineral density. *N Engl J Med.* 2006;354: 821–831.

MacLean C, Newberry S, Maglione M, et al. Systematic review: Comparative effectiveness of treatments to prevent fractures in men and women with low bone density or osteoporosis. *Ann Intern Med.* 2008;148:197–213.

Majumdar SR, Kim N, Colman I, et al. Incidental vertebral fractures discovered with chest radiography in the emergency department: Prevalence, recognition and osteoporosis management in a cohort of elderly patients. *Arch Intern Med*. 2005;165:905–909.

Miller PD, McClung MR, Macovei L, et al. Monthly oral ibandronate theapy in postmenopausal osteoporosis: 1-year results from the MOBILE study. *J Bone Miner Res*. 2005;20:1315–1322.

NIH Consensus development panel on osteoporosis prevention, diagnosis and therapy. Osteoporosis, prevention, diagnosis, and therapy. *JAMA*. 2001;285:785–795.

Tinetti ME, Kumar C. The patient who falls: It's always a trade-off. *JAMA*. 2010;303:258–266.

Wardlaw D, Cummings SR, Van Meirhaeghe J, et al. Efficacy and safety of balloon kyphoplasty compared with nonsurgical care for vertebral compression fracture (FREE): A randomised controlled trial. *Lancet*. 2009;373:1016–1024.

Watts NB. Fundamentals and pitfalls of bone densitometry using dual-energy X-ray absorptiometry (DXA). *Osteoporosis Int*. 2004;15:847–854.

## CHAPTER 8: BACK PAIN IN KIDS: IS IT JUST GROWING PAINS OR IS IT MORE SERIOUS?

Balague F, Troussier B, Salminen JJ. Non-specific low back pain in children and adolescents: Risk factors. *Eur Spine J*. 1999;8:429–438.

Bennett DL, Nassar L, DeLano MC. Lumbar spine MRI in the elite-level female gymnast with low back pain. *Skeletal Radiol*. 2006;35:503–509.

Damborg F, Engell V, Andersen M, et al. Prevalence, concordance, and heritability of Scheuermann kyphosis based on a study of twins. *J Bone Joint Surg Am*. 2006;88: 2133–2136.

Frino J, McCarthy RE, Sparks CY, et al. Trends in adolescent lumbar disc herniation. *J Pediatr Orthop*. 2006;26:579–581.

Kayser R, Mahlfeld K, Greulich M, et al. Spondylodiscitis in childhood: Results of a long-term study. *Spine*. 2005;30:318–323.

Khoury NJ, Hourani MH, Arabi MM, et al. Imaging of back pain in children and adolescents. *Curr Probl Diagn Radiol*. 2006;35:224–244.

Leung AK, Wong BE, Chan PY, et al. Nocturnal leg cramps in children: Incidence and clinical characteristics. *J Natl Med Assoc*. 1999;91:329–332.

Lowe RM, Hashkes P. Growing pains: A noninflammatory pain syndrome of early childhood. *Nature Clin Prac Rheum*. 2008;4:542–549.

Murray PM, Weinstein SL, Spratt KF. The natural history and long-term follow-up of Scheurermann kyphosis. *J Bone Joint Surg Am*. 1993;75:236–248.

Neuschwander TB, Cutrone J, Macias BR, et al. The effect of backpacks on the lumbar spine in children: A standing magnetic resonance imaging study. *Spine*. 2010;35:83–88.

Newton PO, Parent S, Marks M, et al. Prospective evaluation of 50 consecutive scoliosis patients surgically treated with thoracoscopic anterior instrumentation. *Spine*. 2005;30:S100–109.

Pehrsson K, Larsson S, Oden A, et al. Long-term follow-up of patients with untreated scoliosis. A study of mortality, causes of death, and symptoms. *Spine*. 1992;17:1091–1096.

Sponseller PD. Sizing up scoliosis. *JAMA*. 2003;289:608–609.

Watson KD, Papageorgiou AC, Jones GT, et al. Low back pain in schoolchildren: The role of mechanical and psychological factors. *Arch Dis Child*. 2003;88:12–17.

## CHAPTER 9: HOW AND WHEN TO USE
## MEDICATIONS EFFECTIVELY FOR PAIN

Ballantyne JC, Mao J. Opioid therapy for chronic pain. *N Engl J Med*. 2003;349:1943–1953.

Borenstein D. Opioids: To use or not to use? That is the question. *Arthritis Rheum*. 2005;52:6–10.

Chou R, Huffman LH. Medication for acute and chronic low back pain: a review of the evidence for an American Pain Society/American College of Physicians clinical practice guideline. *Ann Intern Med*. 2007;147:505–514.

Elenbaas JK. Centrally acting oral skeletal muscle relaxants. *Am J Hosp Pharm*. 1980;37:1313–1323.

Gimbel J, Linn Hale M, et al. Lidocaine patch treatment in patients with low back pain: Results of an open-label, nonrandomized pilot study. *Am J Ther*. 2005;12: 311–319.

Roelofs PD, Deyo RA, Koes BW, et al. Nonsteroidal anti-inflammatory drugs for low back pain: An updated Cochrane review. *Spine*. 2008;33:1766–1774.

Schnitzer TJ, Gray WL, Paster RZ, et al. Efficacy of tramadol in treatment of chronic low back pain. *J Rheumatol*. 2000;27:772–778.

White WB, West CR, Borer JS, et al. Risk of cardiovascular events in patients receiving Celecoxib: A meta-analysis of randomized clinical trials. *Am J Cardiol*. 2007;99:91–98.

## CHAPTER 10: TREATMENT WITH EXERCISE
## AND PHYSICAL THERAPY

Chou R, Huffman LH. Nonpharmacologic therapies for acute and chronic low back pain: A review of the evidence for an American Pain Society/ American College of Physicians clinical practice guideline. *Ann Intern Med*. 2007;147:492–502.

Elnaggar IM, Nordin M, Sheitchzadeh A, et al. Effects of spinal flexion and extension exercises on low back pain and spinal mobility in chronic mechanical low back pain patients. *Spine*. 1991;16:967–972.

## CHAPTER 11: COMPLEMENTARY THERAPIES

Ashar B, Rowland-Seymour A. Advising patients who use dietary supplements. *Am J Med*. 2008;121:91–97.

Astin JA. Mind-body therapies for the management of pain. *Clin J Pain*. 2004;20:27–32.

Brien S, Prescott P, Bashir N, et al. Systematic review of the nutritional supplements dimethyl sulfoxide (DMSO) and methylsulfonylmethane (MSM) in the treatment of osteoarthrtitis. *Osteoarthritis Cartilage*. 2008;16:1277–1288.

Cherkin DC, Sherman KJ, Avins AL, et al. A randomized trial comparing acupuncture, simulated acupuncture, and usual care for chronic low back pain. *Arch Intern Med*. 2009;169:858–866.

Clegg DO, Reda DJ, Harris CL, et al. Glucosamine chodroitin sulfate and the two in combination for painful knee osteoarthritis. *N Engl J Med*. 2006;354:795–808.

Collacott EA, Zimmerman JT, White DW, et al. Bipolar permanent magnets for the treatment of chronic low back pain: A pilot study. *JAMA*. 2000;283:1322–1325.

Falkenbach A, Oberguggenberger R. Ayurveda in ankylosing spondylitis and low back pain. *Ann Rheum Dis*. 2003;62:276–277.

Flechtner JJ, Brodeur RR. Manual and manipulation techniques for rheumatic disease. *Rheum Dis Clin North Am*. 2000;26:83–96.

Gallagher SP, Romana Kryzanowska R. *The Pilates Method of Body Conditioning*. Philadelphia: Bainbridge Books; 1999:208.

Giordano J. Chronic pain and spirituality: Implications and practical applications for chronic pain management. *Prac Pain Management*. April 2007, 64–66.

Horstman J. Tai chi. *Arthritis Today*. July 2000, 60–62.

Keet L. *The Reflexology Bible*. New York: Sterling; 2008:400.

Lockie A, Geddes N. *The Complete Guide to Homeopathy: The Principles and Practice of Treatment*. London: Dorling Kindersley; 1995:240.

Manheimer E, White A, Berman B, et al. Meta-analysis: Acupuncture for low back pain. *Ann Intern Med*. 2005;142:651–663.

Martel-Pelletier J, Lajeunesse D, Reboul P, et al. Therapeutic role of dual inhibitors of 5-LOX and COX, selective and non-selective non-steroidal anti-inflammatory drugs. *Ann Rheum Dis*. 2003;62:501–509.

Mitchell S. *The Complete Illustrated Guide to Massage*. Boston: Element; 1997:224.

Muller-Fassbender H. Double-blind clinical trial of S-adenosylmethionine versus ibuprofen in the treatment of osteoarthritis. *Am J Med*. 1987;83:81–83.

Trock DH. Electromagnetic fields and magnets: Investigational treatment for musculoskeletal disorders. *Rheum Clin North Am*. 2000;26:51–62.

Williams K, Abildso C, Steinberg L, et al. Evaluation of the effectiveness and efficacy of Iyengar yoga therapy on chronic low back pain. *Spine*. 2009;34:2066–2076.


## CHAPTER 12: WHAT TO KNOW BEFORE YOU CONSIDER SURGERY

Abdu WA, Spratt KF, Tosteson AN, et al. Degenerative spondylolisthesis: Does fusion method influence outcome? Four-year results of the spine patient outcomes research trial. *Spine*. 2009;34:2351–2360.

Boden SD, Balderston RA, Heller JG, et al. Disc replacements: This time will we really cure low back and neck pain? *J Bone Joint Surg Am*. 2004;86:411–422.

Chou R, Baisden J, Carragee EJ, et al. Surgery for low back pain: A review of the evidence for an American Pain Society Clinical Practice Guideline. *Spine*. 2009;34:1094–1109.

Delamarter R. Percutaneous lumbar discectomy, preoperative and postoperative magnetic imaging. *J Bone Joint Surg Am*. 1995;77:578–584.

Freeman BJ, Mehdian R. Intradiscal electrothermal therapy, percutaneous discectomy, nucleoplasty: What is the current evidence? *Curr Pain Headache Rep*. 2008;12:14–21.

Gibson JN, Waddell G. Surgical interventions for lumbar disc prolapse: Updated Cochrane review. *Spine*. 2007;32:1735–1745.

Malmivarra A, Slatis P, Heliovaara M, et al. Surgical or nonoperative treatment for lumbar spinal stenosis? A randomized controlled trial. *Spine*. 2007;32:1–8.

Nierman E, Zakrzewski K. Recognition and management of preoperative risk. *Rheum Dis North Am*. 1999;25:585–622.

Richards JC, Majumdar S, Lindsey DP, et al. The treatment mechanism of an interspinous process implant for lumbar neurogenic intermittent claudication. *Spine*. 2005;30:744–749.

Saal JS, Saal JA. Management of chronic discogenic low back pain with a thermal intradiscal catheter. A preliminary report. *Spine*. 2000;25:382–388.

Shapiro S. Medical realities of cauda equina syndrome secondary to lumbar disc herniation. *Spine*. 2000;25:348–352.

Slipman CW, Shin CH, Patel RK, et al. Etiologies of failed back surgery syndrome. *Pain Med.* 2002;3:200–214.

## CHAPTER 13: LOWER YOUR RISK FOR BACK PAIN WITH PREVENTION: THE ABC PLAN

Andersson GBJ. Epidemiologic aspects on low back pain. *Spine.* 1981;6:53–59.

Cady LD, Bischoff DP, O'Connell ET, et al. Strength and fitness and subsequent back injuries in firefighters. *J Occup Med.* 1979;21:269–272.

Helewa A, Goldsmith CH, Lee P, et al. Does strengthening the abdominal muscles prevent low back pain—A randomizaed controlled trial. *J Rheumatol.* 1999;26:1808–1815.

Kelsey JL, Githens PB, O'Connor T, et al. Acute prolapsed lumbar intervertebral disc. An epidemiologic study with special reference to driving automobiles and cigarette smoking. *Spine.* 1984;9:608–613.

Lahad A, Malter AD, Berg AO, et al. The effectiveness of four interventions for the prevention of low back pain. *JAMA.* 1994;272:1286–1291.

Palmer KT, Syddall H, Cooper C, et al. Smoking and musculoskeletal disorders: Findings from a British national survey. *Ann Rheum Dis.* 2003;62:33–36.

Shiri R, Karppinen J, Leino-Arjas P, et al. The association between smoking and low back pain: A meta-analysis. *Am J Med.* 2010;123:87.e7–35.

## CHAPTER 14: ENJOYING SEX WITHOUT HURTING YOUR BACK

Ambler N, Willaims AC, Hill P, et al. Sexual difficulties of chronic pain patients. *Clin J Pain.* 2001;17:138–145.

Hagg O, Fritzell P, Nordwall A. Sexual function in men and women after anterior surgery for chronic low back pain. *Eur Spine J.* 2006;15:677–682.

Houtchens CJ. Sexual healing. *Arthritis Today.* 1998;(May-June):35–42.

Maigne J, Chatellier G. Assessment of sexual activity in patients with back pain compared with patients with neck pain. *Clin Orthop Rel Res.* 2001;385:82–87.

Rosenbaum TY. Musculoskeletal pain and sexual function in women. *J Sex Med.* 2010;7:645–653.

## APPENDIX A: DR. B'S BACK SCHOOL FAQ

Beurskens AJ, de Vet HC, Koke AJ, et al. Efficacy of traction for nonspecific low back pain: 12-week and 6-month results of a randomized clinical trial. *Spine.* 1997;22:2756–2762.

Hosea TM, Gatt CJ. Back pain in golf. *Clin Sports Med.* 1996;15:37–53.

Kraft CN, Pennekamp PH, Becker U, et al. Magnetic resonance imaging findings of the lumbar spine in elite horseback riders: Correlations with back pain, body mass index, trunk/leg-length coefficient, and riding discipline. *Am J Sports Med.* 2009;37:2205–2213.

Lang AM. Botulinum toxin type B in piriformis syndrome. *Am J Phys Med Rehabil.* 2004;83:198–202.

Watkins RG (ed). The Spine in Sports. St. Louis: Mosby; 1996:1–657.

Yelland MJ, Del Mar C, Pirozzo S, et al. Prolotherapy injections for chronic low back pain: A systematic review. *Spine.* 2004;29:2126–2133.

## APPENDIX B: MEDICATIONS FOR LOW BACK PAIN

*Physicians' Desktop Reference* (www.pdrhealth.com).

# Index

ABC plan, 203–11
acetaminophen, 54, 241–42; dosage and administration of, 130; for fibromyalgia, 92; in pregnancy, 98
active therapies, 221–22
Actonel, 107–8
acupressure, 162
acupuncture, 17, 163–64; definition of, 223
acupuncturist, 31
acute relaxation phase, 140
adalimumab, for spondyloarthropathy, 88
Advil, 55
aerobics, 57–59; machines for, 234
age: and diagnosis, 19; and disc condition, 138; and osteoporosis, 102
AIDS, 83
air mattress, 53
alcohol, 23; and libido, 218; and medications, 125
alendronate, 107; for osteoporosis, 103
Aleve, 55
Alexander, F. Mathias, 172
Alexander technique, 172–73
all-fours position, 216f, 217
allograft, 188–89
alternative therapies. See complementary therapies

amitriptyline, 61, 134–35; for fibromyalgia, 93
Amrix. See cyclobenzaprine
analgesics, 54, 62; definition of, 223; indications for, 121–22
Anaprox. See naproxen
anesthesiologist, 31, 196
aneurysms, 95–96, 232
ankylosing spondylitis (AS), 86; definition of, 223
annulus fibrosis, 10, 10f; definition of, 223
Ansaid, 240
anterior spine surgery, 192
antibiotics: for chlamydia, 87; for discitis, 115
antibody therapies, 136
antidepressants, 61, 134–35; for fibromyalgia, 93; and libido, 218
anti-inflammatory, definition of, 223
anti-inflammatory diets, for spondyloarthropathy, 88–89
anti-inflammatory drugs, xvi; for herniated disc, 72. See also nonsteroidal anti-inflammatory drugs
antioxidants, 208–9
antiseizure drugs, 61, 134; for fibromyalgia, 93
anxiety, 7
applied therapy, 55–57

CBC. *See* complete blood count

CBT. *See* cognitive behavioral therapy

C curve, 148–49, 148*f*; exercises for, 149*f*–151*f*

Celebrex. *See* celecoxib

celecoxib, 125, 240; and surgery, 195

centrology, 167

cervical, definition of, 224

cervical vertebrae, 8

chair: selection of, 206, 230–31; for sex, 217, 217*f*

children: back pain in, 113–19; red flags in, 114–15

chiropractic manipulation, 159–60

chiropractor, 31; selection of, 160–61

chlamydia trachomatis, 86–87

chlorzoxazone, 129, 243

choline magnesium trisalicylate, 241

chondroitin, 178–79

chronic back pain, 60–61; stress and, 94; therapy for, 134–35. *See also* back pain

claudication, 77–78; definition of, 224

Clinoril, 240

closed MRI, 37–39

*clostridium botulinum*, 233

Cobb's angle, 116, 116*f*

coccydynia, 103; definition of, 224

coccyx, 8; definition of, 224

codeine, 132, 241

coffee, and medications, 125

cognitive behavioral therapy (CBT), 170

cold therapy, 55–56; for osteoarthritis, 67

colonic pain, 97

Comfort Zone, 58–59; gradual expansion of, 57–59

communication, on sex, 213–15

complementary therapies, 157–81; precautions with, 158; term, 158; use of, 157

complete blood count (CBC), 46–47

computed axial tomography (CT), 34, 40–41, 41*f*; definition of, 224

conjunctivitis, 86; definition of, 224

contraceptives, oral, for endometriosis, 99

control, versus cure, 61–62

conversion reaction, 6–7; definition of, 224

copper bracelets, 175

corsets, 56–57, 205–6

corticosteroids, 44, 133–35; definition of, 224; epidural injection therapy, 133–34; for fibromyalgia, 92; foraminal injection therapy, 134; for polymyalgia rheumatica, 93–94; side effects of, 133; for spinal stenosis, 79–80

costs of medical tests: bone scan, 43; CT, 40; discography, 44; EMG, 45; MRI, 39; NCV, 45; X rays, 36

counterirritant therapy, 17, 61

COX-2 inhibitors, 123–28; for chlamydia, 87; dosage and administration of, 125–27; precautions with, 125; for spinal stenosis, 79; and surgery, 195

craniosacral massage, 162

C-reactive protein (CRP), 46; definition of, 223

Crohn's disease, 86

crossover leg exercise, 141*f*

cryoablation, 67; definition of, 224

CT. *See* computed axial tomography

cure, versus control, 61–62

cyclobenzaprine, 129, 243; for fibromyalgia, 93; side effects of, 128 cyclooxygenase, 123; definition of, 224

Cymbalta. See duloxetene

Dantrium, 243
dantrolene, 243
Darvocet, 241
Darvon, 241
Daypro, 240
degeneration, 11, 65–69; definition of, 224
Demerol, 242
denosumab, 110
devil's claw, 177
diabetes, 83
diabetic neuropathy, 96
diagnostic tests, 33–47; precautions with, 33–35, 160
diazepam, 129, 243
diclofenac, 124, 240–41
diets: anti-inflammatory, 88–89; bread-free, 90; recommendations, 208–10; vegetarian, 89
diffuse idiopathic skeletal hyperostosis (DISH syndrome), 90–91
diflunisal, 240
digital X ray, 36
Dilaudid, 242
Disalcid, 240
disc(s), 8, 10–11, 10f–11f; artificial, 191; definition of, 224; degeneration of, 11, 65–69, 224; normal variations in, 34; transplants, 199. See also herniated disc
discectomy, 174, 187–88; definition of, 224
discitis, 83; in children, 115; definition of, 224

discography, 43–44; definition of, 224
Discomfort Zone, 58
DISH syndrome, 90–91
diving, 235
doctor: types of, 30–31; working with, 19–31
Dolobid, 240
dowager's hump. See kyphosis
dual energy X ray absorptiometry (DXA), 44, 103; definition of, 224
duloxetene, 61, 136; for fibromyalgia, 93
dura, 14; definition of, 225
Duragesic, 132, 242
DXA. See dual energy X ray absorptiometry

ear acupuncture, 164
Easprin, 240
Ecotrin, 240
education, 158; back school, 229–37; effect of, 59–60, 221–22; resources for, 245–48
Elavil. See amitriptyline
electrodiagnostic tests, 44–46
electromyelography (EMG), 44–45
elimination diets, 89
Embeda, 242
emergency surgery, 191–92
endometriosis, 98–99
endorphins, 17, 214; definition of, 225
epidural, 39; corticosteroid injection therapy, 133–34; definition of, 225; for spinal stenosis, 79
epidural fibrosis, 198–99
epidural lipomatosis, 80
ergonomics, 23; definition of, 225
erythrocyte sedimentation rate (ESR), 46; definition of, 225

ginger, 177–78
GLA. *See* gamma linolenic acid
glucosamine, 178–79
golf, 236–37
golimumab, for
    spondyloarthropathy, 88
growing pains, 113–14
gymnastics, 235

Hahnemann, Samuel Christian, 175
hamstrings, 13; definition of, 225;
    stretching, 142*f*
*Harpagophytum procumbens*, 177
harpagoside, 177
harrington rods, 82
hatha yoga, 165
health care professionals, 30–31
heart failure, 30
heat therapy, 55–56; for
    osteoarthritis, 67
heel lifts, 81
height loss, 102; regaining, 110–11
hemoglobin, 95
herniated disc, 3, 10, 69–71, 69*f*;
    definition of, 226; surgery for,
    73–74; treatment of, 72–73
high heel shoes, 232
high sensitivity C-reactive protein
    (hsCRP), 46
hip, osteoarthritis of, 68–69
Hippocrates, 46
histocompatibility testing, 87–88
history, 19, 23–24
HLA-B$_{27}$, 88
hockey, 235
homeopathy, 175–76
hormone replacement therapy, 106–7
horseback riding, 234–35
hospital stay, 195–96
hot yoga, 166
hsCRP. *See* high sensitivity
    C-reactive protein

human parathyroid hormone,
    109–10
hydrocodone, 132, 242
hydromorphone, 242
hypertension, medications and,
    126–27
hypnosis, 61, 169

ibandronate, 108
IBD. *See* inflammatory bowel disease
ibuprofen, 55, 124, 240
ice massage, 55
IDET. *See* intradiscal electrothermal
    annuloplasty
imipramine, 136
Indocin, 240
indomethacin, 240
infection, 83–84
inflammation, 23; definition of, 226
inflammatory bowel disease (IBD)
    arthritis, 86
inflammatory diseases, 85–90
infliximab, for spondyloarthropathy,
    88
informed consent form, 196
innerspring mattress, 53
instrumentation, spinal, 189–90
internist, 30
interventional radiologist, 31
intervertebral, definition of, 226
intervertebral discs. *See* disc(s)
intradiscal electrothermal
    annuloplasty (IDET), 199
inversion boot therapy, 231–32
iontophoresis, 152–53
iritis, 86
ischemia, 94
isometric flexion exercises, 143–44

jogging, 235
joints, 4; definition of, 226;
    examination of, 29

Kadian, 132, 242
Kegel exercises, 219
ketoprofen, 124, 241
ketorolac, 241
kidney stones, 22–23, 97
knee bend test, 27, 29*f*
knowledge: effect of, 59–60, 221–22; resources for, 245–48
Kryzanowska, Romana, 168
kyphoplasty, 110–11
kyphosis, 24, 25*f*, 102; adolescent, 117–18; brace for, 57; definition of, 226

laminectomy, 187; definition of, 226
lateral bending exercise, 147*f*
leg raise test, 26, 29*f*
leukemia, in children, 115
lidocaine, 127, 241
Lidoderm. *See* lidocaine
lifestyle, and pain, 23
lifting posture, 205–6
ligaments, 4, 12; definition of, 226
ligamentum flavum, 76
limbrel, 178
Lioresal, 243
lipomatosis, epidural, 80
Lodine, 240
lordosis, 20, 87; definition of, 226; in pregnancy, 97–98
Lortab, 242
low back, definition of, 226
low back pain. *See* back pain
lumbar, 4; definition of, 226
lumbar discs, 8
lumbar spine: anatomy of, 4, 5*f*, 8; examination of, 24–25
lumbar spondylosis, 65–69
lumbar vertebrae, 8
lymph nodes, 4
Lyrica, for fibromyalgia, 93

magnetic resonance imaging (MRI), xv, 33, 37–40, 38*f*; definition of, 226; open versus closed, 37–39; precautions with, 34–35
magnets, 17, 173–75
maintenance therapy, 160
manipulation, 59–60, 158–61; definition of, 226
Margin Zone, 58
massage, 17, 162; ice, 55
massage therapist, 31
mattresses, types of, 53
McKenzie, Robin, 144
mechanical back pain, 3–4; recognition and treatment of, 63–82
meclofenamate, 240
Meclomen, 240
medical back pain, 3–5; in children, 114–15; recognition and treatment of, 83–99
medical disorders, red flags of, 4
medical history, 19, 23–24
medications, 121–36, 239–43; indications for, 121–22; information packet with, 233; interactions with, 174–75; and libido, 218–19; over-the-counter, 54–55, 124; postoperative, 196; for spondylosis, 66
meditation, 165, 171
mefanamic acid, 241
meloxicam, 240
men: and osteoporosis, 104–5. *See also* sex differences
menstruation, and back pain, 98–99
meperidine, 242
meridians, 162–63
metaxalone, 129, 243
methadone, 242
methocarbamol, 243
methylsulfonylmethane, 180

orphenadrine, 129, 243
orthopedic surgeon, 30; selection of, 193–94
Orudis. *See* ketoprofen
Oruvail. *See* ketoprofen
osteoarthritis, 65–69; chondroitin and glucosamine for, 178–79; definition of, 227; of hip, 68–69; treatment of, 67–68
osteomyelitis, 83
osteopathic manipulation, 161
osteophytes, 76
osteoporosis, 19, 101–11; definition of, 227; diagnosis of, 104; lifestyle and, 23; prevalence of, 101; prevention of, 105–10; risk factors for, 102–3
over-the-counter medications, 54–55, 124
oxaprozin, 240
oxycodone, 72, 132, 242
OxyContin, 132, 242
oxymorphone, 242

pain: definition of, 16; factors affecting, 21–22; location of, 20–21; nerves and communication of, 14–16; quality and intensity of, 22–23; sex differences in, 16; timing of, 20, 22
pain management practitioner, 31
pain threshold, fluctuation in, 16–17
Pamelor, 136
Parafon. *See* chlorzoxazone
parathyroid hormone, 109–10
paresthesias, 77
Patanjali, 165
patient controlled analgesia (PCA), 196
pelvic tilt, 215; in standing position, 143*f*

Pennsaid, 241
Percocet, 242
Percodan, 242
percutaneous discectomy, 187–88
personal trainer, versus physical therapist, 138
physiatrist, 30
physical activities: controlling, 51–52; postoperative, 196–97
physical examination, 24–30
physical therapist, 31; versus personal trainer, 138; working with, 137–39
physical therapy, 137–55; benefits of, 138; evaluation for, 138–39; postoperative, 197
Pilates, Joseph, 167
Pilates Method, 167–68
pillowtop mattress, 53
piriformis syndrome, 26, 74
piroxicam, 240
placebo, 157; definition of, 227
polymyalgia rheumatica (PMR), 93–94
Ponstel, 241
pool exercises, 153–54
posterior longitudinal ligament (PLL), 12
postoperative period, 196–97
posture, 204, 204*f*; and back pain, 3; lifting, 205–6; sitting, 206; standing, 206; stretching, 206–7
pranayama, 165
prednisone, 72, 133–35; for polymyalgia rheumatica, 93–94; for spinal stenosis, 80
pregabalin, 134; for fibromyalgia, 93
pregnancy, and back pain, 97–98
preoperative evaluation, 194–95
prevention, 203–11
progesterone, 106–7

S curve, 148–49, 149f; exercises for, 149f–151f
seat supports, 230
seizures, 61
selective estrogen receptor modulator (SERM), 107, 111; definition of, 228
selective serotonin reuptake inhibitors (SSRIs), for fibromyalgia, 93
semi-Fowler position, 52
septic arthritis, 83
SERMs, 107, 111; definition of, 228
sertraline, 136; for fibromyalgia, 93
sex, 213–20; exercises for, 219; positions for, 215–17, 216f–217f
sex differences: and diagnosis, 19; and osteoporosis, 101–2, 104–5; in pain, 16; in sacroiliac joints, 9–10
sex therapist, 220
shiatsu, 162
shoes, 232
sickle cell disease, 95
sitting posture, 206
sit-ups, partial, 142f
Skelaxin. See metaxalone
skiing, 235–36
sleep positions, 52
slipped disc. See herniated disc
smoking, 23; abstaining from, 203–4; and medications, 125; and surgery, 195
snow shoveling, 64
Soma. See carisoprodol
spacers, 192–93
spasm, 63–65; treatment of, 128
spinal cord, 8, 14; definition of, 228
spinal cord stimulator, 198
spinal inflammatory arthritis. See spondyloarthropathy

spinal instrumentation, 189–90
spinal stenosis, 21, 76–81; definition of, 228; differential diagnosis of, 77–78; surgery for, 80–81; treatment of, 79–80, 133
spine, curves of, 8, 9f
spine spacers, 192–93
spondylitis, 86
spondyloarthropathy, 20, 85–86; in children, 115; definition of, 228; finding, 87–88; treatment of, 88–90
spondylolisthesis, 35, 75–76, 75f; adolescent, 118–19; definition of, 228
spondylosis, 65–69, 75–76; definition of, 228; treatment of, 66
spoon position, 216f, 217
sports: golf, 236–37; horseback riding, 234–35; selection of, 235–36
squat test, 27, 29f
SSRIs. See selective serotonin reuptake inhibitors
standing posture, 206
stationary bicycle, 234
stenosis. See spinal stenosis
Still, Andrew Taylor, 161
straddle position, 216f, 217
strain, 35, 63–65; definition of, 228
strengthening phase, 146
stress, yoga for, 165–66
stretching posture, 145, 206–7
structural integration, 162–63
subluxations, 159
sulindac, 240
surgery, 183–200; emergency, 191–92; failed, 197–99; future of, 199; for herniated disc, 73–74; indications for, 186; postoperative period, 196–97;

websites, on back pain, 245–47
weight loss, 210; for spinal stenosis, 80
Welsh, Tom, 148
Williams, Paul, 143
women: hormone replacement therapy for, 106–7; menstruation and back pain, 98–99; pregnancy and back pain, 97–98. *See also* sex differences
work: and pain, 23; persistence in, 210–11; seating for, 231
World Health Organization, on osteoporosis, 104

Xodol, 242
X ray, 6, 33; conventional, 35–36, 36*f*; definition of, 228; precautions with, 34–35, 160

yoga, 61, 165–66; definition of, 228

Zachrisson-Forssell, Marianne, 229
Zanaflex, 243
*Zingiber officinale,* 177–78
zoledronic acid, 108
Zoloft. *See* sertraline
Zorprin, 241
Z score, 103

# About the Author

David Borenstein, M.D., is clinical professor of medicine and former medical director of the Spine Center at the George Washington University Medical Center. Dr. Borenstein is a board-certified internist and rheumatologist who is internationally recognized for his expertise in the care of patients with back pain and spinal disorders.

Dr. Borenstein received his undergraduate degree from Columbia University in 1969. His medical school, internal medicine residency, and rheumatology fellowship training were completed at the Johns Hopkins University Medical School and Hospital from 1969 to 1978. He became an assistant professor of medicine at the George Washington University Medical Center in 1978. He was promoted to professor of medicine in 1989. He became a clinical professor of medicine on the voluntary faculty in 1997.

Dr. Borenstein is an author of a number of medical articles and books, including *Low Back Pain: Medical Diagnosis and Comprehensive Management* (2nd ed.). This book has been recognized by the Medical Library Association Brandon/Hill list as one of the two hundred essential books for a medical library. He is also author of *Neck Pain: Medical Diagnosis and Management*. Both of these books were combined to be published as *Low Back and Neck Pain: Comprehensive Diagnosis and Management* in 2004. He has lectured to the general public on behalf of the Arthritis Foundation on a variety of medical topics. He has chaired low back pain symposia for a number of physician groups, including the American College of Rheumatology. He has also moderated national telesymposia sponsored by pharmaceutical companies for physicians and has served as a medical guest expert for CNN, CBS, and local news programs.

Dr. Borenstein is a fellow of the American College of Physicians and American College of Rheumatology. He is a member of the International Society for the Study of the Lumbar Spine and is listed in *The Best Doctors in America* since 2000. He has served as a guest expert for the Food and Drug Administration, Arthritis Advisory Board Conference on Acute and Chronic Pain. He is included in *Who's Who in Medicine and Healthcare*, *Who's Who in America*, and *Who's Who in the World*. He is in active clinical practice in Washington, D.C.

About the Author